"This refreshing book notes that trauma emerges from the subjective *response to the event*, rather than the event itself. This is the first book to extend beyond traditional frontline professions to include others that are also vulnerable to trauma and traumatic reactions. As a result, the book is an extraordinary and lucid overview of the field from the perspective of trauma and posttraumatic growth."

Charles R. Figley, PhD, *the Tulane University Paul Henry Kurzweg, MD, distinguished chair in Disaster Mental Health and director of the Tulane University Traumatology Institute*

"Internationally-known researcher Jane Shakespeare-Finch has teamed up with an extensive range of interdisciplinary colleagues to produce this important collection. This is a beautifully organized book that follows the journeys of emergency first responders to those who remain involved long after the immediate situation averts, and it combines personal vignettes with rigorous reviews of the literature. It will serve as a welcome resource to students, academics, and practitioners alike."

Professor Cheryl Regehr, *vice president and provost, University of Toronto*

"This book makes an invaluable contribution to the literature on resilience and posttraumatic growth. There are similarities but also distinct differences among the various groups of frontline workers. Each chapter provides a unique understanding of posttraumatic growth that is greatly needed not only to facilitate health and wellness in the individual, but also to improve our overall society. I highly recommend the work of these authors."

Professor Brian A. Chopko, PhD, PD, *Department of Sociology and Criminology, Kent State University at Stark*

Trauma, Resilience, and Posttraumatic Growth in Frontline Personnel

Trauma, Resilience, and Posttraumatic Growth in Frontline Personnel examines the history, context, nature, and complexity of working in front-line services. Chapters provide a detailed overview of specific mental health models that are applicable both on a day-to-day basis and to disaster and major event response. The book also details elements of mental health responses that have been proven to facilitate coping, minimize risk, and promote both resilience and posttraumatic growth. These strategies include, but are not limited to, peer support programs, mental health education, and psychological first aid. Each chapter incorporates research on PTSD, anxiety, and depression as well as research relating to posttraumatic growth, resilience, connectedness, and belongingness.

Trauma, Resilience, and Posttraumatic Growth in Frontline Personnel is a vital guide for those who provide care to trauma survivors as well as for researchers and scholars.

Jane Shakespeare-Finch has spent 25 years conducting research to inform psychoeducation and intervention programs promoting resilience and posttraumatic growth in frontline personnel.

Paul J. Scully has worked in emergency services for over 40 years, first as a paramedic, then paramedicine educator, and later as a clinical psychotherapist.

Dagmar Bruenig works in genetics and epigenetics maintaining a focus on interdisciplinary research. Dagmar has worked with diverse cohorts, including military personnel, paramedics, and correctional services officers.

The Routledge Series in Posttraumatic Growth

Richard G. Tedeschi and Bret A. Moore
Series Editors

The Routledge Series in Posttraumatic Growth includes authored and edited texts that identify and distill the most relevant information for students, practitioners, researchers, organizational leaders, and policy makers in the areas of psychological health, wellness, and growth. Volumes in the series focus primarily on concepts that guide discovery, development, and implementation of interventions that increase psychological strength and flexibility, facilitate health and recovery, and support responses of individuals, communities, and institutions in times of adversity and trauma.

Trauma, Resilience, and Posttraumatic Growth in Frontline Personnel
Edited by Jane Shakespeare-Finch, Paul J. Scully, and Dagmar Bruenig

Trauma, Resilience, and Posttraumatic Growth in Frontline Personnel

Edited by

Jane Shakespeare-Finch, Paul J. Scully
and Dagmar Bruenig

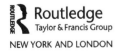

NEW YORK AND LONDON

Designed cover image: stereohype © Getty Images

First published 2024
by Routledge
605 Third Avenue, New York, NY 10158

and by Routledge
4 Park Square, Milton Park, Abingdon, Oxon, OX14 4RN

Routledge is an imprint of the Taylor & Francis Group, an informa business

Library of Congress Cataloging-in-Publication Data
Names: Shakespeare-Finch, Jane, editor. | Scully, Paul J., editor. |
Bruenig, Dagmar, editor.
Title: Trauma, resilience, and posttraumatic growth in frontline personnel /
edited by Jane Shakespeare-Finch, Paul J. Scully and Dagmar Bruenig.
Description: New York, NY : Routledge, 2024. |
Series: Routledge series in posttraumatic growth |
Includes bibliographical references and index. |
Identifiers: LCCN 2023038779 (print) | LCCN 2023038780 (ebook) |
ISBN 9781032268934 (hardback) | ISBN 9781032268927 (paperback) |
ISBN 9781003292807 (ebook)
Subjects: LCSH: Post-traumatic stress disorder–Treatment. |
Psychic trauma–Treatment. | Posttraumatic growth. | Resilience (Personality trait) |
First responders–Mental health services. | First responders–Mental health.
Classification: LCC RC552.P67 T7554 2024 (print) |
LCC RC552.P67 (ebook) | DDC 616.85/21–dc23/eng/20231211
LC record available at https://lccn.loc.gov/2023038779
LC ebook record available at https://lccn.loc.gov/2023038780

ISBN: 9781032268934 (hbk)
ISBN: 9781032268927 (pbk)
ISBN: 9781003292807 (ebk)

DOI: 10.4324/9781003292807

Typeset in Janson MT Std
by Newgen Publishing UK

This book is dedicated to all the frontline and high-risk workers who, day after day, work to keep individuals and communities safe. No words can describe the immense gratitude we have for your work and the impact you have on the well-being of people and communities around the world. Thank you!

Contents

Foreword

It is with great satisfaction that I introduce you to the first volume in *The Routledge Series on Posttraumatic Growth and Resilience*. This initial volume is a fitting start for this series as it is edited by my great friend and colleague, Jane Shakespeare-Finch, who is as well-informed as anyone in the world about the concept of posttraumatic growth. She has been studying posttraumatic growth for over 20 years and made major contributions to its measurement and application, especially in the context of the experiences of public safety personnel. Her co-editors for this volume are very gifted and well informed on the concepts of posttraumatic growth and resilience. Paul Scully has been in the trenches for many years working with ambulance service personnel, developing and delivering programs to meet their mental health needs. He knows the price they pay for their work that we all depend upon in our times of greatest need, and has been dedicated to their support. Developing programs to promote posttraumatic growth and resilience demands cultural competence, that is, knowing the experience of the people you serve. Paul has an extraordinary degree of cultural competence. Dagmar Bruenig has been developing a remarkable program of research on biomarkers of PTSD, resilience, and posttraumatic growth. This work indicates the epigenetic mechanisms involved in trauma experience, and deepens our understanding of the challenges to healthy functioning in people exposed to trauma at various times in their lives. Her work on the physiological effects of childhood trauma and occupational trauma helps us to appreciate the challenges faced by many first responders, and those who are developing programs to assist them in becoming more resilient.

Jane, Paul, and Dagmar have assembled an experienced and knowledgeable group of authors for the chapters in this volume. Each has a deeply personal connection to the work of people in frontline occupations. This is reflected in the tone of empathy and admiration in each of these chapters. The occupations discussed in this volume are emergency medical dispatchers, law enforcement officers, firefighters, paramedics, disaster and emergency response professionals and volunteers, emergency nurses and physicians, child protection workers, humanitarian aid workers, correctional officers, mental health care professionals, and military service members. The editors have also included chapters that provide a concise and current examination of the topics discussed in the chapters on each of the frontline occupations. This allows readers who are looking to understand posttraumatic growth and resilience concepts to learn the basics and find where to go for more information.

I encourage readers of this volume to focus on the book as a whole, and to not restrict themselves to particular occupational groups that they are most interested in serving. This is because the ideas and programs described in each chapter can translate to other occupations very well. All the occupations here have much in common, as the people in them are often motivated by a desire to serve, some personal meaning or experience that is behind this motive, a willingness to tolerate stress and loss, and too often a lack of support from their own organizations or communities that is reflected in low pay, long hours, and lack of equipment. In this volume, one of the greatest needs of these personnel is addressed: effective mental health care.

Despite the challenges faced by public safety personnel, reports of posttraumatic growth are commonplace, and the authors of the chapters in this volume describe for us how this growth is experienced, and the impact of it on the personnel, and by extension, the people they serve. Most importantly, we also find descriptions of how posttraumatic growth can be facilitated and supported. The posttraumatic growth process is a pathway to resilience, so that the future traumas that are inherent in the work of these occupations can be managed with a perspective that allows workers to continue to serve in ways that meet the needs of their communities without sacrificing their own mental wellness.

The occupations represented here are often highly regarded. This respect can come at a price, however. Among the general public, and often among those working in the occupations, there can be a false assumption of superhuman strength that makes front-line workers immune to the terrible and frequent stresses of their work. This can contribute to a lack of resources devoted to mental health support, or a lack of willingness to make use of the resources available. The stigma and shame associated with help-seeking is one of the greatest obstacles to wellness in these professions.

Even those workers in occupations that have garnered much respect in the past do not always receive as much support now. For example, I have spoken with many in the medical professions who have endured disrespect and suspicion during the COVID-19 pandemic. Some patients have villainized them for their support of vaccines, their insistence on quarantine measures, or their inability to save their loved ones. This has been a very demoralizing experience for many of these health care workers. This kind of treatment is an additional burden for those whose work life is already stressful.

Some occupations in this volume have always suffered from a lack of consideration and respect. Among these I would suggest are the child protection workers, correctional facility staff, human remains recovery and identification workers, and emergency dispatchers. Their work is not as often recognized or in the public eye. Therefore, less public recognition and support for their organizations creates additional stress for these personnel. For readers unfamiliar with the work of these people, the chapters that describe it will be enlightening.

In this volume there is also much to offer those who manage the organizations that employ and support front-line emergency workers. These managers are crucial in providing safe psychological environments for their employees, so that they have no shame or stigma to contend with when seeking the support they will inevitably need during their careers. The authors of these chapters discuss what effective support can be so that those who design and manage organizations can revisit their programs and improve them. They should do so while recognizing that posttraumatic growth should be foremost in their designs.

Trauma is inevitable in these professions, obviously. Resilience is never going to be perfected, so that people are not affected by these experiences or recover without struggle. Given the inevitable struggles, posttraumatic growth provides a sense of meaning and purpose to these experiences, and compassion for oneself and others. With posttraumatic growth, there is more recognition that the natural, human responses to the tragedies of frontline work no longer need to be viewed as symptoms of disorder. That when this challenging work stirs up pain from childhood, it is a possible route to healing childhood trauma. That being in this work can result in the deepest connections to coworkers and the people being served. Being in this work can yield the most profound understanding of what it means to face death head on, and by doing so, to live a human life fully, with wisdom, and with gratitude.

Richard Tedeschi, Ph.D.
Boulder Crest Institute for Posttraumatic Growth
Bluemont, VA, USA

Table

Abbreviations

ACEM	(Australasian College for Emergency Medicine)
ACEP	(Australian College of Emergency Physicians)
AM	(Antemortem)
APA	(American Psychiatric Association)
ASD	(Acute Stress Disorder)
CASCW	(Center for Advanced Studies in Child Protection)
CBT	(Cognitive Behavioral Therapies)
CDC	(Centers for Disease Control and Prevention)
CISD	(Critical Incident Stress Debriefing)
COs	(Correctional Officers)
CPT	(Cognitive Processing Therapy)
DASS	(Depression, Anxiety, and Stress)
DP	(Depersonalization)
DRB	(Distress Reduction Behaviors)
DSM-5	(Diagnostic and Statistical Manual of Mental Disorders, Fifth Edition)
EDs	(Emergency Departments)
EE	(Emotional Exhaustion)
EMDR	(Eye Movement Desensitization and Reprocessing)
EMDs	(Emergency Medical Dispatchers)
EMS	(Emergency Medical Services)
EPs	(Emergency Physicians)
ESG	(Environmental, Social, and Government)
FKBP5	(FK506 Binding Protein 5)
FSB	(Financial Stability Board)
HW	(Humanitarian Workers)
ICD-11	(International Classification of Disease-11)
LE	(Law Enforcement)
LEO	(Law Enforcement Officers)
MACSSA	(Minnesota Association of County Social Service Administrators)
MDD	(Major Depressive Disorder)
MFI	(Mass-fatality Incidents)
MST	(Military Sexual Trauma)

NET	(Narrative Exposure Therapy)
NR3C1	(Nuclear Receptor Subfamily 3 Group C Member 1)
PA	(Personal Accomplishment)
PFA	(Psychological First Aid)
PM	(Post-mortem)
PMR	(Proportionate Mortality RatioPSO (Peer Support Officer)
PPE	(Personal Protective Equipment)
ProQOL	(Professional Quality of Life)
PTE	(Potentially Traumatic Events)
PTG	(Posttraumatic Growth)
PTGI	(Posttraumatic Growth Inventory)
PTSD	(Posttraumatic Stress Disorder)
RCT	(Randomized Controlled Trial)
STS	(Secondary Traumatic Stress)
TCFD	(Taskforce on Climate-related Financial Disclosures)
TIC	(Trauma-informed Care)
UN	(United Nations)
UNDRR	(United Nations Office for Disaster Risk Reduction)
UNHCR	(United Nations High Commissioner for Refugees)
USAID	(United States Agency for International Development)
vPTG	(Vicarious Posttraumatic Growth)
WHO	(World Health Organization)

About the Contributors

Kaye Adams, B.B.Sc. (Hons-Psych), served for 15 years in the Royal Australian Navy including operational deployments to Iraq. After leaving the military in 2007, she has specialized in mental health services for trauma, incarcerated youth, and domestic and family violence. After registering as a psychologist in Australia, Kaye has worked extensively in clinical roles with first responders, veterans support services, and military personnel, in addition to several roles as the national manager for not-for-profit military veteran psychology services.

Dagmar Bruenig, Ph.D., is an Early Career Academic at the School of Biomedical Sciences, QUT. During her PhD, Dagmar investigated genetic and psychological predisposition to risk and resilience to PTSD in military veterans, being the first researcher to investigate resilience as a psychological construct rather than disorder absence in molecular research. Dagmar has a keen interest in the broad variations in post-trauma responses with a particular focus on resilience. Having worked in genetics and epigenetics for seven years, she maintains a focus on interdisciplinary research that combines differentiated approaches to understanding psychological constructs. Dr Bruenig has been working across different frontline cohorts, such as military personnel, paramedics, and correctional services officers.

James Douglas, B.B.Sc; G.Dip.App.Psych is a psychologist with nearly two decades of experience working with emergency service organizations, specifically in State Emergency Services (SES). James has a particular interest in how people prepare for, and respond to, high impact events and how organizations might use the science of psychology to invigorate wellbeing and resilience and maximize performance. Whether it is clinical frameworks, neuropsychology, organizational development strategy, psychological assessment, or process consultation, James is curious about how the evidence might be a guide to an enriched, safer, and more productive workplace. He is co-director of the THRIVE Institute and is currently working with helicopter pilots to build a comprehensive wellbeing program for their Helicopter Rescue & Emergency Medicine pilots, crew, engineers, staff, and their families.

Peter Ellis, M.D., is a forensic pathologist. He has a special interest in Disaster Victim Identification (DVI) and has participated in many incidents around the world. Peter was the lead Australian pathologist for the Tsunami response in 2004, managing the Australian pathology operation, and has worked in several offshore DVI programs including the Bali bombing, air crashes in Nepal and Papua New Guinea, as well as the Christchurch, New Zealand earthquakes. He has conducted many DVI training programs in South East Asia as well as in Australia. He has also worked in Kosovo, East Timor and Sri Lanka and has an active interest in identification science, especially after disasters and mass grave excavations. He was the consulting forensic pathologist to the WWI Fromelles mass grave project in northern France. He is the Chair of the Interpol DVI Pathology/Anthropology Sub-Working Group and is the sole pathologist advising Interpol on DVI matters.

Mohamed Elshazly, M.D., is a consultant psychiatrist from Egypt with more than 15 years of experience in clinical mental health services, capacity building, and humanitarian mental health programs in Egypt, Turkey, Iraq, and Bangladesh. Since February 2018, he has been working in Cox's Bazar, Bangladesh, as the mental health and psychosocial support officer with UNHCR, the refugee agency of the United Nations. In this role, Mohamed is responsible, with his team, for mainstreaming mental health interventions within the humanitarian response, particularly in health and protection, strengthening of community based mental health initiatives, and scaling up brief psychological interventions. Prior to his deployment to Bangladesh, Mohamed worked with UNHCR in the Kurdistan Region of Iraq for two years (2016–2018), with International Medical Corps in the Middle East (2013–2016), Psycho-Social Services and Training Institute Cairo (PSTIC), and Doctors Without Borders in Egypt (2012–2013).

Gerald Fitzgerald, M.D. is an Emeritus Professor of Public Health and discipline Leader of Health Management and Disaster Management. He holds medical specialist qualifications in Emergency Medicine and Medical Administration and has previously held positions as the Director of an Emergency Department, Medical Director and then Commissioner of the Queensland Ambulance Service followed by being the States Chief Health Officer. His principal research focus is on emergency healthcare systems and how they perform under both routine and nonroutine pressures. He has published over 150 peer reviewed articles, a text in Disaster Health Management, eight book chapters and more than 100 conference representations. He has supervised more than 30 PhD students to completion and obtained over $5m in research grants.

Megan Fry, B.Psych (Hons). M.Clin.Psych. is a clinical psychologist who owns and operates a private practice in Queensland, Australia. As an ex-serving soldier and military Psychologist in the Australian Army, Megan has spent her career working with military personnel (current serving and ex-serving). As an Advanced Individual Schema Therapist, Megan has developed a unique schema therapy approach when working with military personnel, which has resulted in improved clinical outcomes in the therapy room and which she is currently further investigating in her research at the School of Applied Psychology, Griffith University.

Leanne Hinsch, B.Psych. (Hons), is a psychologist, co-founder, and co-director of the THRIVE Institute of Performance & Wellbeing. For 28 years Leanne has worked across both organizational and clinical domains designing, implementing, and managing growth-focused psychological wellbeing, safety, and performance systems; peer support, leadership and staff preparedness, and resilience programs; high impact event response management frameworks; trauma treatment, performance recovery, and human optimization practices; safety authority regulation support; and the development, training and supervision of a national trauma-informed counselling and coaching network of psychologists and mental health professionals in Australia. These services are provided with safety-critical high-performance industries supporting emergency aeromedical, medical, aviation, airline, military, policing, and human service industries.

K.C. Kalmbach, Ph.D., is an Associate Professor of psychology and licensed clinical psychologist. Over the past two decades, she has held positions as a researcher, administrator, clinician, consultant, and educator. Before joining the faculty at Texas A&M University-San Antonio, Dr. Kalmbach worked with colleagues to help build the first juvenile offender mental health court in Houston, Texas. Prior to this, as faculty at California State University-Los Angeles, she conducted community needs assessments for the Los Angeles Mayor's Office of Gang Reduction/ Youth Development (GRYD). Before entering academia, Dr. Kalmbach served as a director of the Texas Regional Center for Policing Innovation, a federally funded training institute tasked with providing progressive training for law enforcement and justice system personnel. Currently, in addition to teaching, she provides clinical consulting to a range of agencies and organizations including law enforcement and the military. Her research and publications to date center around ethico-legal issues, moral injury, and posttraumatic growth.

Robyn Kirby, B.B.Sc. (Hons-Psych) is a registered Psychologist and researcher with a specialization in trauma within Emergency Service organizations. Robyn's experience spans over 25 years working with private and public sector agencies, where she has led and implemented a range of organizational mental health initiatives, including management of critical incident services, disaster support response, and peer support programs. Robyn combines her academic research with direct leadership experience in supporting emergency service teams to deliver quality services tailored to address evolving needs. She is inspired by the selfless dedication of her fire service colleagues and strives to continually improve the support services for emergency service staff, volunteers, and their families.

Gülşah Kurt, Ph.D. is a Clinical Psychologist from Türkiye with experience in mental health and the integration of immigrants. She is currently a Postdoctoral Research Fellow at the University of New South Wales (UNSW), Australia. She did her Ph.D. on mental health and integration of asylum seekers and refugees in Türkiye. Her current research focuses on the resilience and well-being of asylum-seeking communities in low and middle-income countries and high-income countries.

Emma Malone, M.Clin. is a Clinical Psychologist who has 15 years clinical experience working with people who have experienced trauma, primarily with people who have experienced complex/developmental trauma. She currently works as a clinical psychologist and child and family therapist in a specialist trauma service that provides therapy to children and adults who have experienced child abuse, neglect, and domestic violence. In her time working in complex trauma, Emma has held both case management and therapeutic roles in a number of trauma specific organizations including child protection services and sexual abuse counselling programs. In addition, Emma provides consultation and supervision around working with people who have experienced complex trauma, including being a member of the advisory committee for the Australian Law Reform Commission's inquiry into the Family Law system. Emma is currently completing her Ph.D. research looking at the embodied expressions of vicarious trauma in therapists.

Ellyse McCormick, R.N. is a Clinical Research Nurse and registered Midwife. Elly began her career in infectious diseases before spending time in the UK, living, working, and travelling. She has worked as an emergency nurse and is now a clinical researcher with a special interest in wellness, stress and coping in emergency service personnel. Elly is currently undertaking her Master of Public Health and has been awarded a nationally competitive grant to undertake a research project in stress and coping in emergency staff. In her spare time, Elly enjoys travel, snowboarding, photography, and spending time with family.

Olivia Miller, B.B.Sc. (Hons-Psych), is a doctoral student at the Queensland University of Technology in the School of Psychology and Counselling. Her Ph.D. is examining the wellbeing of Custodial Correctional Officers using a salutogenic framework. She has a keen interest in understanding post-trauma responses, particularly posttraumatic growth, and promoting wellbeing in high-risk groups. Her previous work in this area has included understanding epigenetic risk and protective factors for post-trauma outcomes, including posttraumatic growth in paramedicine students; and understanding factors that support the health and wellbeing of Disaster Victim Identification workers for the National Institute of Forensic Science.

Louise Munro, Ph.D., is a counselling psychologist in private practice who has a 30-year career spanning nursing, mental health, counselling, and clinical supervision as a registered psychologist and registered nurse. For the last ten years Louise has been lead academic in a Master of Counselling program teaching from a philosophical position that privileges a social constructionist framework, making visible alternative explanations and amplifying hidden competence. Through the use of therapeutic teams, people are supported to examine existing narratives and create new narratives that better fit their life experiences. This style of therapeutic work offers opportunities to look at the experience of trauma through multiple lenses and invites new and unique perspectives to support growth, adjustment, and processes of meaning making for clients and therapists. Work life balance means juggling academic work private practice, a beautiful family, and two Italian greyhounds.

Gillian Ray-Barruel RN, Ph.D., is a conjoint Senior Research Fellow in the Griffith University School of Nursing and Midwifery and Queen Elizabeth II Jubilee Hospital, Brisbane, Australia. Following a successful and rewarding 15-year career as a critical care nurse in Brisbane and New York, Gillian engaged her passion for English literature and completed a doctorate in the field of literary disability studies. She has now established a career as an internationally respected nurse researcher, focusing on improving assessment and decision-making by bedside clinicians to prevent patient complications and improve healthcare outcomes. After identifying a gap between evidence-based guidelines and clinical practice, she created the I-DECIDED® device assessment and decision tool, which is now used in many hospitals worldwide. When she's not writing and presenting, Gillian enjoys reading, creative writing, and spending time on the coast with her family and Golden Retriever.

Olga Rebolledo, M.Soc.Dev.Psych., is a Colombian psychologist with more than 15 years of experience in mental health and psychosocial programming. Olga has set up and implemented national programmes in Colombia, Bangladesh, South Sudan, and Nigeria. Olga has extensive experience in designing tools and protocols to integrate psychosocial approaches within humanitarian responses as well as designing mechanisms to improve capacity of the Strengthening Mental Health through Psychological Support (MHPSS) response.

Simon Rosenbaum, Ph.D. is an Associate Professor and Scientia Fellow in the School of Psychiatry, University of New South Wales, Sydney, and an honorary fellow at the Black Dog Institute. As an exercise physiologist, Simon's research focuses on physical activity, mental illness, sport for development, and global mental health. Simon has worked with a variety of groups including youth, veterans, emergency service workers, and refugees. Simon has published >170 peer-reviewed publications including a textbook. He serves as an elected national director of Exercise and Sports Science Australia and is President of the Australasian Society for Traumatic Stress Studies. Simon has led international research and capacity building projects, including with the United Nations migration agency (IOM) working in the Rohingya refugee crises in Bangladesh. In 2019, Simon was recognized by the Clarivate Highly Cited list for mental health, awarded to the top 1% of researchers worldwide, based on citations.

Benjamin J. Ryan, Ph.D., MPH, is from Baylor University, USA. Ben has experience working, researching, and teaching in environmental health science, communicable and noncommunicable diseases, community resilience, global health, humanitarian assistance, and disaster risk reduction. He has led activities in these fields across the Indo-Pacific, Europe, and North America. His field experience includes environmental health assessments in city and rural settings, responses to natural disasters and disease outbreaks, mass casualty incidents, failures of critical business functions, managing projects in Indigenous communities and facilitating delivery of health services to asylum seekers. He has worked at local, state, and federal levels of government in Australia and the United States. Ben has also published numerous peer-reviewed articles, guidelines, book chapters and conducted media interviews relating to disaster management and environmental health science.

Paul J. Scully, M.Couns., is a Clinical Psychotherapist. He is the founder and inaugural manager of the Staff Support "Priority One" Mental Health and Peer Support program within the Queensland Ambulance Service (QAS), Australia. Prior to this, Paul spent many years as a paramedic and then as a paramedic educator. Paul has been a Visiting Fellow and Adjunct Associate Professor at the Centre for Disaster and Emergency Medicine at the Queensland University of Technology (QUT) Australia. He has co-facilitated mental health research projects and has published and co-authored articles and book chapters relating to mental health and coping within the ambulance service work setting. He has played a key role in the development of workplace mental health and peer support programs for a large range of organizations in Australia including St John Ambulance Northern Territory and Ambulance Service Tasmania, as well as having been a workplace mental health consultant to international ambulance organizations including the Scottish, London, and Northumbria Ambulance Services in the UK.

Jane Shakespeare-Finch, Ph.D., is Professor in the School of Psychology and Counselling at Queensland University of Technology (QUT), Australia. Jane's primary area of teaching is psychological trauma, and her primary area of research is in posttraumatic growth. Starting her research with emergency service personnel 25 years ago, Jane continues to work with emergency services in the promotion of positive post-trauma outcomes and has also investigated the construct of trauma, post-trauma adaptation and posttraumatic growth in various populations including survivors of sexual assault, natural disasters, bereavement, and refugees. Jane is currently working to create novel approaches to trauma research in transdisciplinary teams looking at a range of post-trauma outcomes using epigenetics, EEG, and neurofeedback methods. Recent projects also include working with the Queensland Corrective Services, the Australian Federal Police, and the Office of Justice and Attorney General. Jane is Immediate Past President of the Australasian Society for Traumatic Stress Studies, is on the editorial board of two international journals, and is a Scientific Advisory Board member for the Boulder Crest Institute for Posttraumatic Growth in the USA. Professor Shakespeare-Finch has enjoyed supervising more than 80 post-graduate student theses and has published approximately 150 peer-reviewed works.

Vivienne Tippett Ph.D., MPH, OAM has been the Director of Research for the School of Clinical Sciences at QUT since 2013. She is the past Director of the Australian Centre for Prehospital Research and has extensive experience as a researcher and consultant to government in the emergency pre-hospital, disaster health and emergency health systems. Her work has been recognized with a Medal of the Order of Australia (OAM) for services to medical education (2018) and a Distinguished Service medal from Queensland Ambulance Service (2012) for services to paramedic research. She is a Fellow of the Jamieson Trauma Institute and was Lead Researcher for the Warnings and Communication Theme of the Bushfire and Natural Hazards CRC (2013–2021). This research program was recognized with a Cooperative Research Centre Association national award for research innovation (2019). Her research has been published in numerous peer-reviewed journals and book chapters.

Renée Treolar-Munro, D.CP. (Clin), is a clinical psychologist and the executive manager for Psychological Education for the Queensland Ambulance Service (QAS). She has a 20-year history working with the QAS in various HR, psychology, and staff support roles, and also works in private practice. Dr Treolar-Munro completed her doctoral thesis assessing the psychological wellbeing of ambulance officers and has been actively involved in a range of ambulance workplace reforms. Notable contributions include her work with the Council of Ambulance Authorities to collaborate and develop best practice recommendations around the recruitment of ambulance officers across many different job roles, and more recently, delivering improvements to the allocation and availability of psychology sessions, clinical utility of information, and ensuring best practice therapeutic approaches continue to be offered to ambulance personnel and their families. Dr Treloar-Munro has a special interest in trauma informed care focusing on prevention of psychological injury, salutogenesis, and posttraumatic growth.

Howard Way, O.B.E. is a mass fatalities management and Disaster Victim Identification (DVI) specialist. He has over 30 years' experience within law enforcement working for London's Metropolitan Police and the United Kingdom National Disaster Victim Identification Unit. Howard has significant experience in managing or supporting the response to mass fatalities operations globally. He is a member and past Chair of the INTERPOL DVI Working Group and chair of the London Mass Fatalities Working Group. He has delivered DVI training, workshops, and mass fatalities capacity building projects in over 20 countries. In 2015 he was honored by HM Queen Elizabeth II for services to Disaster Victim Identification.

Ruth Wells, Ph.D., is a Research Fellow in the Trauma and Mental Health Unit in Psychiatry and Mental Health at the University of New South Wales, Sydney, Australia. Their research focuses on improving MHPSS service provision in humanitarian settings globally and bringing to light how conflict and social exclusion can impact on the well-being of displaced communities. They bring a feminist and decolonizing lens to critically evaluate mental health services towards being more person-centred, equitable. and inclusive. They have a strong commitment to participatory research practices and are humbled to have the opportunity to work together with Syrian, Turkish, and Bangladeshi colleagues, as well as people from refugee backgrounds living in Australia.

Mental Health Strategies within Frontline Organizations

part I

Introduction, Core Concepts, and Purpose

Jane Shakespeare-Finch

Who are Frontline, High-Risk Personnel?

Historically, occupations that are referred to as frontline workers have been primarily comprised of law enforcement services, fire departments, ambulance or prehospital care services, and disaster rescue personnel. But with increased research focusing on mental health in occupational settings over recent decades, it is has become apparent that the term "frontline workers" needs to be broadened to include other occupations as well. This is because there is a wide range of professional and voluntary roles that put people in a position where they are at a comparatively elevated risk for exposure to potential trauma. Although this text is not exhaustive in its coverage of such occupations and voluntary roles, academics, frontline personnel, and practitioners have come together to discuss the impacts of trauma, the likelihood of resilience, and the potential for PTG in 14 frontline occupations or settings. Sometimes the authors, as can be seen in the biographies presented earlier, fill multiple roles; for example, as a paramedic and a psychotherapist, or as a military veteran and a clinical psychologist. The occupations included in this text are emergency medical dispatchers, law enforcement officers, firefighters and paramedics, disaster and emergency response professionals and volunteers, emergency nurses and physicians, child protection workers, humanitarian aid workers, correctional officers, mental health care professionals, and the military.

Prevalence of Mental Ill-Health

So why the need for such a text? Frontline workers are at increased risk of experiencing highly challenging and potentially traumatic events in the line of their duties. Much research has shown that prevalence rates for mental health issues such as posttraumatic stress disorder (PTSD), depression, and anxiety are higher in frontline and emergency response professions than in the general population, hence the term "high-risk". For example, in a large-scale study of police and emergency responders

DOI: 10.4324/9781003292807-2

in Australia, Beyond Blue (2018) found significantly higher rates of psychopathology: in some cases groups were nine times more likely to have a psychiatric disorder, when compared to normative data from the general population. Kindermann et al. (2020) found much higher rates of psychopathology in German emergency call takers and dispatchers. Petrie et al. (2018) conducted a meta-analysis of studies with paramedics and found an overall prevalence rate of psychopathology at 27%. A study by Jyothindran et al. (2021) examining the mental health of emergency physicians in the United States claimed 54% of physicians had burnout and Finnegan and Randles (2022) found psychiatric disorder in the UK military to be common. Obviously, psychopathology can have devastating impacts for the individual and their loved ones, but in these occupations, it can also have serious implications for organizations and the community more broadly. Experiencing PTSD, depression, anxiety, burnout, and other debilitating ways of being can have a negative impact on the worker and their family but pragmatically, also on decision making, memory, concentration, and the overall execution of the person's work-related duties.

Trauma

It is arguably because of the negative impact of trauma, such as those noted above, that disciplines like medicine, psychology, counseling, and other allied health professions are trained in the psychopathology of trauma, if indeed they have any training in trauma at all. Reflecting its pathogenic origin, the word trauma comes from the Greek *troma*, meaning wound or pierce. Although originally a term used to refer to the physical impact and manifestations of a wound, as time has moved on, we have learned that trauma has emotional, cognitive, and behavioral impacts; that the mind and body are inextricably bound. As van der Kolk has written about for some decades now (e. g., 1996; 2014), trauma leaves an imprint on your brain, your body, and your mind. It impacts the individual, but also society more broadly.

There are many texts about the history of trauma, the evolution of understanding for millennia to the current day, and the array of potential consequences of exposure. Therefore, we do not provide that level of detail here. However, it is important to understand the standpoint taken about what trauma is in this text. That is, the position we take is that it is not necessarily the nature of an event that constitutes trauma so much as it is the person's response to an event; their subjective perception. As Judith Herman states, "traumatic events overwhelm the ordinary systems of care that give people a sense of control, connection and meaning … Traumatic events overwhelm the human adaptation to life" (1992, p. 33). That is to say, for an experience to be deemed traumatic, rather than potentially traumatic, it is initially overwhelming. It is an experience that leads people to question their assumptions about the world and who they are in it, and manifests in ways such as producing unwanted thoughts or images, hyperarousal, and avoidance of situations or reminders of the trauma (Tedeschi et al., 2018).

Pathogenesis

Trauma tends to be viewed through a lens of pathogenesis. Pathogenesis literally translates from Greek as "the origins of suffering". Like trauma, historically the term has been primarily linked to the physical – to pathogens that are able to cause disease. And like trauma, it is now used to describe diseases or disorders that impact the mind and brain. It is also the theoretical lens with which health professionals are trained. Indeed, when a person or persons are suffering, alleviating suffering becomes a primary objective. Disentangling psychiatric disorders and finding effective ways of symptom reduction is a core focus of all helping disciplines. However, it is not the only way to think about mental health, although it is an effective way of thinking about mental ill-health.

Salutogenesis

In more recent years, for some people, including the editors and many authors who have contributed to this text, the focus on mental ill-health has shifted towards a more holistic view of mental health in frontline workers. This approach recognizes that while negative sequalae from traumatic experiences exist, positive outcomes such as resilience or post-traumatic growth are more prevalent than lasting pathology. This theoretical lens is called salutogenesis, a term coined by Aaron Antonovsky in the latter half of the 20th century (1979; 1996). Salutogenesis literally translates to "the origins of health", a combination of Greek and Latin roots. Unlike pathogenesis which dichotomizes health as a person being either healthy or ill, salutogenesis views health on a continuum that is influenced by many factors such as the sociocultural and historical context, disease, conflict, stress, politics, pollutants, and religion. Where a person lies on the health-ease/dis-ease continuum is influenced by these factors and the person's sense of coherence.

The sense of coherence refers to a person's capacity for comprehensibility, manageability, and meaningfulness related to a particular event or experience; that an experience can be comprehended, a faith in oneself that they can manage the experience and have the capacity to make sense or bestow meaning to the experience. It is a generalized and long-lasting sense of confidence that a person has the resources to meet demands so that things will generally work out (Antonovsky, 1979). A strong sense of coherence thus implies a person generally has the resources to meet demands but does not suggest that a person will not have ups and downs in their life. If working from a pathogenic framework a clinician may focus on a deteriorating sense of coherence, whereas a salutogenically-oriented clinician would focus on strengthening a person's sense of coherence through setting achievable goals and highlighting internal and external strengths. Two further concepts used throughout this text, that fit well within a salutogenic theoretical framework, are resilience and posttraumatic growth.

Resilience

Resilience has been variously defined as both a trait and state concept. That is, it has been defined as a personality trait and related to concepts such as hardiness (Maddi, 2013). Alternatively, it has been defined as a state. In other words, resilience as a response to a particular event or experience. In this sense resilience is a person's capacity to bounce back or bounce forward (Bonanno, 2005; Masten, 2019). In trying to predict trauma trajectories, including PTSD, recovery, and delayed onset PTSD, resilience has been consistently found to be the most common trajectory following exposure to potential trauma (e. g., Bonanno, 2005; Bonanno et al., 2012). Unlike recovery, after a mild disruption in what is normal functioning for the person, resilient people quite quickly assess the potentially traumatic situation they are in to be manageable and return to pre-event levels of functioning.

After many years studying resilience and factors that relate to or predict resilient outcomes, Bonanno (2021) draws attention to what he calls the resilience paradox. What he is referring to is that following decades of research to identify factors that predict resilience, from personal characteristics, coping strategies, and resources to emotional regulation and context, empirical studies have failed to adequately come up with models that reliably predict resilience. There have, however, been some interventions and psychoeducation programs in emergency services that have provided evidence that resilience, and mental health more generally, can be enhanced. These programs are covered in more detail in Chapter 2, and subsequent chapters in this text. Regardless, when it comes to defining resilience, both of these conceptualizations of resilience are related to the sense of coherence concept as a belief that things will generally work out and are also related to the concept of posttraumatic growth (Almedom, 2007; Ragger et al., 2019).

Posttraumatic Growth

Posttraumatic growth (PTG) is a term coined by Professors Tedeschi and Calhoun in the mid-1990s. It refers to positive changes a person, or community, may perceive following the experience of trauma. Positive changes do not occur as a by-product of exposure but rather as a result of the struggle that is engaged in to integrate the experience into a revised narrative encompassing the experience (Tedeschi et al., 2018). This is likely the result of considerable work including deliberate effortful rumination, restructuring of schemas, finding meaning, and creating a new narrative. Often negotiating such a journey is helped with the assistance of a trusted other, someone to disclose to, to share with and receive support. Calhoun and Tedeschi (2006) used the term "expert companion" to describe such a person. The person need not be a mental health professional; they may be a peer, a trusted family member or friend. The expert companion model is discussed further in Chapter 2.

As far as measurement is concerned, the Posttraumatic Growth Inventory (PTGI) (Tedeschi & Calhoun, 1996) and subsequent versions measure 5 factors: Positive changes in relating to others, appreciation of life, personal strength, changes in priorities and religious, spiritual or existential changes. The various PTG inventories have been found to be reliable and valid in diverse cultural contexts, albeit sometimes with a different factor structure. For example, the newer Posttraumatic Growth Inventory – Expanded (PTGI-X) has been administered in more than a dozen countries and found to be reliable and valid (Taku et al., 2021; Tedeschi et al., 2017). The factor structure of the original and short-from PTGI (Tedeschi & Calhoun, 1996) has been replicated in cultures as diverse as Australia (Morris et al., 2005); Italy (Prati & Pietrantoni, 2014); Pakistan (Aslam & Kamal, 2019); and Iran (Heidarzadeh et al., 2017). Yet in some research, factor structures have differed such as the PTGI (1996) eliciting a single factor structure in South Korea (Yi & Kim, 2014) and a different solution again in Japan (Taku et al., 2007).

Since its origins in the 1990s PTG has been extensively researched in a variety of front-line work settings, enabling this research to inform and enhance the benefits of proactive mental health support strategies. The first published paper in the emergency service context demonstrated that PTG was much more prevalent than symptoms of PTSD (Shakespeare-Finch et al., 2003). More recently Wu and colleagues (2019) reported PTG in the moderate to high range in high-risk occupations. As PTG has become a focused element in contemporary research within frontline work settings, it has highlighted several critical related elements including resilience, connectedness, and organizational belongingness. These factors are discussed throughout the text relative to particular occupations or settings. Overall, they provide guidance to organizations to implement a variety of mental health strategies which embrace a range of needs and that are proactively facilitated, enhancing the confidence and security of employees.

Another important concept in PTG is that if a person perceives they have experienced PTG, it does not discount the very real experience of trauma and distress that was the catalyst for PTG. Further, it does not imply that there is not intermittent ongoing distress. In other words, PTG and distress or symptoms of PTSD can coexist (Tedeschi et al., 2018). Research has found mixed results about the nature of this relationship, with some suggesting a positive linear relationship and others a negative linear relationship. However, a meta-analysis of 42 studies that measured both PTG and symptoms of PTSD revealed that although there was a positive linear relationship, a curvilinear relationship accounted for more variance (Shakespeare-Finch & Lurie-Beck, 2014).

How the Text is Structured

Chapter 1, to this point, has outlined key concepts and theoretical underpinnings that feature throughout this text and has provided a rationale supporting the need for such a resource. Chapter 2 focuses on the necessity for organizations to embrace appropriate guidance and leadership in the application of effective education and training to support employee mental health. It highlights that the burden of responsibility falls upon employers to ensure that not only are mental health resources and strategies in place prior to employment and deployment, but also ongoing focused support, counselling, and other resources are available at all times. Psychoeducation is not limited to frontline personnel. It is imperative that supervisors and managers are sufficiently trained to monitor and facilitate intervention strategies as required.

Emergency call takers and dispatchers are often the first people who are alerted to a crisis. Therefore, they are first occupation examined in Chapter 3. Although not physically on the frontline, emergency dispatches have a very high cognitive load. When someone calls an emergency line, it is because they are in a state of crisis. The call taker has to use tremendous skill to extract information about the nature of the crisis, location, and what is needed, often also trying to use the person as a tool at the scene (e. g., to perform CPR), as well as locating and dispatching an appropriate response crew.

In Chapter 4, law enforcement personnel are the focus. Although the law enforcement officer role can include mundane aspects, it also elevates levels of exposure to potentially traumatic experiences. Like other roles included in this text, law enforcement officers may experience trauma directly, for example as the victim of a physical assault, and indirectly, bearing witness to the trauma of others.

Paramedics or ambulance officers are responsible for attending to medical emergencies and providing necessary pre-hospital care. This occupational group are the focus in Chapter 5. The rates of exposure to trauma and to vicarious trauma in this group are very high given that they only respond to medical emergencies including cardiac arrests, suicides, sudden infant death syndrome, and severe road trauma. Coupled with an innate desire to save lives and assist people in critical need of medical care, paramedics are vulnerable to the impacts of trauma. In this chapter research also attests to the capacity of paramedics to experience elevated levels of PTG and that in most cases they are resilient to the trauma they face.

The third group of what were traditionally referred to as emergency responders (police, paramedics, fire), are the firefighters examined in Chapter 6. The role of a firefighter differs in certain jurisdictions. What firefighters around the world have in common is of course fighting fires, but what differs is that in some countries firefighters are also trained emergency medical responders, some carry the jaws of life so attend to road accidents, some are professional and many more are volunteers whose levels of training vary greatly. There are also a variety of specialist roles such as those who are charged with containing toxic waste or are forensic investigators responsible for identifying factors that contributed to a fire.

Chapter 7 is dedicated to the many thousands of people who are volunteer disaster and rescue personnel. Often volunteers are paid professionals in an allied area such as police, fire, or ambulance services and others are simply committed members of a community. There are unique challenges for volunteers that are discussed in this chapter. Some of those unique challenges relate to the amount of training, resources, and funding available to them. Sometimes the only responders to an emergency, for example in rural and remote areas, are volunteers. This means that often the person or people in need of help are known to them. A personal connection or being in a situation of shared trauma can intensify an already intense experience.

During COVID-19 the role of nurses as frontline personnel was in the forefront of the community's mind. Of course, they have always been frontline personnel, including those nurses who work in emergency departments, palliative care, and in mental health wards. Chapter 8 is dedicated to exploring the role of nurses, the unique challenges of their role and the complex systems and context in which they work. The chapter includes a section about nurses during COVID-19, highlighting the massively increased pressure they were under and how this has impacted their mental health and decision about staying in their work role. The chapter also highlights the need for systemic and comprehensive organizational support structures and resources.

Emergency physicians are a specialist group of medical personnel who, as their title suggests, are the medical leaders in emergency departments and essentially the frontline of the hospital system. In Chapter 9 the complexity of this role is examined as well as the complexity of the context in which they work.

Another complex working environment is correctional facilities or prisons. Like some other professions, such as police and fire, literature makes it clear that there is a hesitancy in these work roles for people to admit to having challenges regarding their mental health and consequently, there is a stigma associated with seeking support when needed.

In Chapter 10 this issue of stigma and the associated 'macho-culture' in prisons is discussed as it acts as a barrier to communicate about mental health, engage in support programs, and subsequently may reduce the chances to develop resilience and PTG.

Chapter 11 examines factors implicated in the high rates of mental ill-health and increasing numbers of suicides, primarily in military veterans. The authors explain indoctrination into the military and how this shapes identity which acts as a source of strength, protection, and camaraderie when serving, and also how it can lead to difficulties following service. They highlight some of the effective programs that have been developed to assist in transition for this group.

Child protection workers are highly trained in their fields to work with children and families, but often do not receive sufficient training in common aspects of the role such as dealing with trauma and domestic violence. Chapter 12 explores these issues and others that are pertinent for this frontline role such as the cumulative impact of constant exposure to child abuse and neglect. Child protection workers have increasing workloads as more and more children are coming into care with complex needs, caseloads are increasing, and turnover in the system is high. Yet, through supportive trauma-informed organizational structures, excellence in supervision, and processing of work-related trauma, these frontline workers are able to build resilience and, for some, experience PTG.

Chapter 13 discusses trauma, resilience, and PTG in mental health professionals. Through careful listening to other's stories and empathetic engagement, mental health professionals are also vulnerable to vicarious trauma and burnout and concurrently afforded the opportunity for vicarious PTG as they bear witness to the growth of their clients. The chapter focusses on integrative approaches to therapy and highlights the important role of supervision for people in this occupation.

Unlike most chapters in this text, Chapter 14 provides a unique insight into a particular work context rather than a single profession. The chapter details working in the context of human remains identification services; people who attend to scenes around the world following mass-fatality disasters. Personnel come from many different professions, for example forensic pathologists, doctors, nurses, dental experts, police, paramedics, legal and administrative fields. The chapter outlines the unique challenges of working in mass fatality contexts which are, by their nature sudden, far reaching and "always stressful." The authors, who have both spent many years in the field, also speak of the comfort they take in providing closure for families when remains have been identified.

Another group of people who are mixed in their discipline backgrounds and work roles are the humanitarian workers discussed in Chapter 15. The contexts in which they work are usually perilous and in low-income settings and/or areas of conflict, including war. Hence, resources are generally scarce, trauma is often palpable and ongoing. Despite the complexities they face and the trauma they are exposed to, the chapter also identifies the rewarding components of the role and the potential for PTG.

In Chapter 16 the topic is counselling frontline personnel. There is a need to understand the context in which frontline personnel operate, the unique stress and trauma they face directly and indirectly as they bear witness to the suffering of others and do what they can to help alleviate that suffering. No-one, regardless of how well they are trained, is immune to the effects of stress and trauma when they work in frontline occupations. Therapeutic alliance and safety are maximized when the therapist can demonstrate an understanding of the context in which their client operates. Not only does this help guide therapeutic sessions but also promotes confidence in the frontline worker that it is safe to share the intimate details of their stories.

In Chapter 17 the focus is on community recovery rather than a particular occupation. The chapter highlights social and systemic resources needed for collective PTG and discusses ways in which communities may become more resilient following shared trauma such as natural disasters. The final chapter in this text summarizes the book, drawing threads of commonality together and explicating differences faced in these unique roles and work contexts. Chapter 18 also discusses the cultural relativity of concepts covered. Although trauma, resilience, and posttraumatic growth are universal concepts, the research reviewed herein also points to some differences in the way that these concepts are abstracted and ways in which they may manifest individually and socially. Essentially, Chapter 18 is about a summary and reflection on the content of the text.

References

Almedom, A. M. (2007). Resilience, hardiness, sense of coherence and posttraumatic growth: All paths leading to "light at the end of the tunnel? *Journal of Loss and Trauma, 10,* 253–265. doi:10.1080/15325020590928216

Antonovsky, A. (1979). *Health, Stress and Coping.* Jossey-Bass

Antonovsky, A. (1996). The salutogenic model as a theory to guide health promotion. *Health Promotion International, 11,* 11–18. doi:1093/heapro/11.1.11

Aslam, N., & Kamal, A. (2019). Assessing positive changes among flood affected individuals: Translation and validation of the post-traumatic growth inventory – sort form (PTGI-SF). *Pakistan Journal of Medical Research, 58,* 59–65. Retrieved from http://pjmr.org.pk/

Bonanno, G. A. (2005). Resilience in the face of trauma. *Current Directions in Psychological Science, 14,* 135–138. doi:10.1111/j.0963-7214.2005.00347.x

Bonanno, G. A. (2021). The resilience paradox. *European Journal of Psychotraumatology, 12.* doi:10.1080/20008198.2021.1942642

Bonanno, G. A., Kennedy, P., Galatzer-Levy, I. R., Lude, P., & Elfström, M. L. (2012). Trajectories of resilience, depression, and anxiety following spinal cord injury. *Rehabilitation Psychology*, *57*, 236–247. doi:10.1037/a0029256

Beyond Blue (2018). *Answering the Call. National Survey on Police and Emergency Services.* Accessed at www.beyondblue.org.au

Calhoun, L. G., & Tedeschi, R. G. (2006). Expert Companions: Posttraumatic Growth in Clinical Practice. In L. G. Calhoun & R. G. Tedeschi (Eds.), *Handbook of posttraumatic growth: Research & practice* (pp. 291–310). Lawrence Erlbaum Associates Publishers

Finnegan, A., & Randles, R. (2022). Prevalence of common mental health disorders in military veterans: using primary healthcare data. *BMJ Military Health*. doi:10.1136/bmjmilitary-2021-002045

Heidarzadeh, M., Naseri, P., Shamshiri, M., Dadkhah, B., Rassouli, M., & Gholchin, M. (2017). Evaluating the factor structure of the Persian version of the posttraumatic growth inventory in cancer patients. *Asian Nursing Research*, *11*, 180–186. doi:10.1016/j.anr.2017.07.003

Herman, J. (1992). *Trauma and recovery: The aftermath of violence – from domestic abuse to political terror.* Perseus Books

Jyothindran, R., d'Etienne, J. P., Marcum, K., Ho, A. F., Robinson, R. D., Tijerina, A., Graca, C., Knowles, H. C., Zenarosa, N. R., & Wang, H. (2021). Association between burnout and wellness culture among emergency medicine providers. *Clinical and Experimental Emergency Medicine*, *8*, 55–64. doi:10.15441/ceem.20.074

Kindermann, D., Sanzenbacher, M., Nagy, E., Greinacher, A., Cranz, A., Nikendei, A., Friederich, H. C., & Nikendei, C. (2020). Prevalence and risk factors of secondary traumatic stress in emergency call-takers and dispatchers – a cross-sectional study. *European Journal of Psychotraumatology*, *11*, 1799478. doi:10.1080/20008198.2020.1799478

Maddi, S. (2013). Personal Hardiness as the Basis for Resilience. In: Hardiness: Turning stressful circumstances into resilient growth, 7–17. Springer Briefs in Psychology. Springer.

Masten, A. S. (2019). Resilience from a developmental systems perspective. *World Psychiatry*, *18*, 101–102. doi:10.1002/wps.20591

Morris, B. A., Shakespeare-Finch, J., Rieck, M., & Newbery, J. (2005). Multidimensional nature of posttraumatic growth in an Australian population. *Journal of Traumatic Stress Studies*, *18*, 575–585

Petrie, K., Milligan-Saville, J., Gayed, A., Deady, M., Phelps, A., Dell, L., Forbes, D., Bryant, R., Calvo, R., Glozier, N., & Harvey, S. (2018). Prevalence of PTSD and common mental disorders amongst ambulance personnel: a systematic review and meta-analysis. *Social Psychiatry & Psychiatric Epidemiology*, *53*, 897–909. doi:10.1007/s00127-018-1539-5

Prati, G., & Pietrantoni, L. (2014). Italian adaptation and confirmatory factor analysis of the full and short form of the posttraumatic growth inventory. *Journal of Loss and Trauma*, *19*, 12–22. doi:10.1080/15325024.2012.734203

Ragger, K., Hiebler-Ragger, M., Herzog, G., Kapfhammer, H. P., & Unterrainer, H. F. (2019). Sense of coherence is linked to post-traumatic growth after critical incidents in Austrian ambulance personnel. *BMC Psychiatry, 19.* doi:10.1186/s12888-019-2065-z

Shakespeare-Finch, J., & Lurie-Beck, J. (2014). A meta-analytic clarification of the relationship between posttraumatic growth and symptoms of posttraumatic distress disorder. *Journal of Anxiety Disorders, 28,* 223–229. doi:10.1016/j.janxdis.2013.10.005

Shakespeare-Finch, J., Smith, S. G., Gow, K. M., Embelton, G., & Baird, L. (2003). The prevalence of post-traumatic growth in emergency ambulance personnel. *Traumatology, 9,* 58–71. doi:10.1177/153476560300900104

Taku, K., Calhoun, L. G., Tedeschi, R. G., Gil-Rivas, V., Kilmer, R., & Cann, A. (2007). Examining posttraumatic growth among Japanese university students. *Anxiety, Stress and Coping, 20,* 353–367. doi:10.1080/10615800701295007

Taku, K., Tedeschi, R. G., Shakespeare-Finch, J., Krosch, D., David, G., Kehl, D., Grunwald, S., Romeo, A., di Tella, M., Kamibeppu, K., Soejima, T., Hiraki, K., Volgin, R., Dhakal, S., Zięba, M., Ramos, C., Leal, I., Nunes, R., Gouveia, P., Tomás, C., Del Prado Chaves, P., Senol-Durak, E., Canevello, A., Cann, A., & Calhoun, L. G. (2021) Posttraumatic Growth and Posttraumatic Depreciation across Ten Countries: Global Validation of the PTG-PTD Theoretical Model. *Personality and Individual Differences, 169.* doi:10.1016/j.paid.2020.110222

Tedeschi, R. G., & Calhoun, L. G. (1996). The posttraumatic growth inventory: Measuring the positive legacy of trauma. *Journal of Traumatic Stress, 9*(3), 455–471.doi:10.1002/jts.2490090305

Tedeschi, R. G., Cann, A., Taku, K., Senol-Durak, E., & Calhoun, L. G. (2017). The posttraumatic growth inventory: A revision integrating existential and spiritual change. *Journal of Traumatic Stress, 30,* 11–18. doi:10.1002/jts.22155

Tedeschi, R. G., Shakespeare-Finch, J., Taku, K., & Calhoun, L. G. (2018). *Posttraumatic Growth: Theory, Research and Applications.* New York, NY: Routledge

van der Kolk, B., McFarlane, A. C., & Weisaeth, L. (1996). *Traumatic stress: The effects of overwhelming experience on mind, body and society.* The Guilford Press

van der Kolk, B. (2014). *The body keeps the score: Mind, brain and body in the transformation of trauma.* UK: Penguin Random House

Wu, X., Kaminga, A. C., Dai, W., Deng, J., Wang, Z., Pan, X., & Liu, A. (2019). The prevalence of moderate-to-high posttraumatic growth: A systematic review and meta-analysis. *Journal of Affective Disorders, 243,* 408–415. doi:10.1016/j.jad.2018.09.023

Yi, J., & Kim, M. A. (2014). Postcancer experiences of childhood cancer survivors: How is posttraumatic stress related to posttraumatic growth? *Journal of Traumatic stress, 27,* 461–467. doi:10.1002/jts.21941

Psychoeducation, Leadership, and Interventions

2

Jane Shakespeare-Finch and Paul J. Scully

Employer's Obligation to Promote and Support Staff Mental Health

As highlighted by McDiarmid and colleagues (2021), frontline workers, such as those in healthcare, have always had a duty of care to their patients. But organizations also have a duty of care to their employees. This is particularly true for those in frontline and high-risk occupations and people who work in high-risk contexts. Extending beyond the moral and ethical responsibility of organizations to do all they can to protect and promote the health and wellbeing of their staff, there is also a legal precedence to provide psychoeducation and support to staff and people in positions of authority need to be able to identify if their staff or volunteers are struggling, specifically where there is a foreseeable risk (Freckelton, 2008).

Education, Training, and Health Promotion

Evidence-informed recommendations for high-risk organizations in managing mental health attest that organizations should provide a broad range of support services to meet diverse needs, with a stepped care approach that extends support and treatment as needs escalate and a trauma-informed care (TIC) approach (Kim et al., 2021; Phoenix Australia, 2020). A stepped process involves the collaborative and coordinated support of leaders, trained Peer Support Officers (PSOs), professional counsellors, and organizational policy and procedures to "activate" avenues for psychosocial support (Beyond Blue, 2018; Cherry et al., 2021; Creamer et al., 2012; Phoenix Australia, 2020). TIC shares many of these features and also puts an onus on the organization to create a culture of TIC. To date, frontline organizations have been inconsistent in their adoption of TIC, with some doing it better than others (Kim et al., 2021).

Psychological preparedness is one of the variables found to improve wellbeing and increase resilience in frontline personnel, which provides a strong rationale for the importance of training

DOI: 10.4324/9781003292807-3

and education (Shakespeare-Finch, 2007). Although there are some common factors, the most effective programs are targeted for specific audiences, address specific needs of the work-role, encourage early access to seek assistance, and are continually offered (e.g., to new recruits, experienced frontline workers, tailored for specialist roles or high-risk groups, and in preparation for retirement). There may also be specific programs following major incidents or organizational change. Training and support for leaders, managers and supervisors is a high priority to raise awareness of mental health and increase understanding of their valuable role in mitigating psychosocial risk and building a resilient workforce (Cook & Mitchell, 2013; WHO, 2022). Beyond safety requirements, organizations can go a step further to build a culture that creates opportunity for posttraumatic growth to occur (Tedeschi et al., 2018).

Risks are generally managed through effective systems and embedded processes which identify and address potential psychological risks. Adopting a salutogenic approach, organizations may also aim to incorporate strategies and initiatives that foster resilience and promote posttraumatic growth rather than solely focusing on the reduction of symptoms of psychopathology. The framework of support is to raise mental health awareness in individuals, supervisors, and managers; identify issues early; engage in open discussion about mental health concerns; and maintain awareness of support options (Beyond Blue, 2018; WHO, 2022). This framework also embraces the need for organizational connectedness and for trust and safety within organizations, the promotion of organizational and individual connection (Shakespeare-Finch & Daley, 2017). It is important to also highlight that confidentiality is crucial to the success and reputation of support services (Scully, 2011).

Social support and a sense of organizational belongingness are key factors in supporting and addressing workplace well-being. Research has highlighted that workers report higher levels of resilience when they feel valued and supported in the workplace (Shakespeare-Finch & Daley, 2017). With the benefit of research, formally trained Peer Support Officers (PSOs) have also been shown to be a significant resource for mental health support in front line settings (Cherry et al., 2021; Feuer, 2021; Scully, 2011). Using a Delphi technique, Creamer and colleagues (2012) conducted research with experts around the world that provided a detailed model of what constitutes a comprehensive PSO program with the best chance of it being effective. Unfortunately, most organizations follow some, but not all, of the guidelines provided. Psychosocial support through PSO programs, mentors, and regular opportunities for people to socially connect has significant benefits for mental health and wellbeing in these work settings (Feuer, 2021; WHO, 2022). The positive influence of a broader social support system, such as family and friends external to the organization, has also been recognized (Beyond Blue, 2018; Tedeschi et al., 2018).

Interventions in Frontline Occupations

While an entire book could be dedicated to pro-active, reactive, and maintenance programs to support and promote mental health in frontline personnel, here we highlight key elements of successful programs, and review three programs that have an evidence base in frontline contexts. Other programs are discussed throughout the text. As stated earlier, the best interventions are tailored to the context which is most effectively done through participatory research with the targeted population and intervention experts. However, evidence-based interventions have not always been the expectation. An early strategy well known within most frontline work settings was Critical Incident Stress Debriefing (CISD), which became part of a broader Critical Incident Stress Management model. The approach was formally promoted in a text published by Mitchell and Everly (1995), based on Mitchell's background as a paramedic and firefighter and Everly's background as a psychologist in the USA. CISD was administered shortly after exposure to trauma in a group setting following a particular manualized protocol, in some cases by certified facilitators. Whilst this approach was introduced and promoted extensively and applied following a variety of both high-level events and following "smaller" low profile incidents in emergency services, research has revealed its limitations. For example, Rose and colleagues (2002) conducted a meta-analysis of CISD research and found it to be benign at best and toxic in some circumstances. More research has been conducted since and more calls have been made to cease the CISD practice in another review (Burchill, 2019) and more broadly (WHO, 2019) including in frontline organizations (Feuer, 2021). Hence, almost all frontline work settings no longer use the approach. The failure of this intervention highlighted the need for rigorous evaluation of approaches prior to them being adopted widely.

Therefore, strategies for providing effective primary interventions for frontline organizations in the form of psychoeducation and comprehensive staff support services became an urgent focus. Much work has been conducted over recent decades to ensure such programs are tailored to the work role and context, and some programs have been subjected to rigorous independent evaluation to ensure their effectiveness in promoting mental health and buffering mental ill-health. We outline three of these programs below but firstly, there are some commonalities in recommendations. The first strategy is that psychoeducation starts at the stage of recruitment and/or in vocational training if that is required for the profession. This includes ensuring that employees are aware of the potential impacts on mental health as a result of the challenges that are inherent in their work. Strategies involve teaching about what the signs and symptoms of psychological difficulty are, encouraging reflection and self-care, and ensuring that personnel know how to access confidential and professional support when needed (Beyond Blue, 2022; WHO, 2022).

Another aspect is to ensure that education is ongoing and fit for purpose as with ongoing education and skill development related to the specific work setting. Organizations cannot rely on teaching personnel something once. There should be ongoing education, similar to professional development, that is updated as new evidence comes to light. By fit for purpose, we mean that often employees move to different roles. For example, you may be a trained paramedic or police officer who moves into a management role. Being an effective worker on the frontline does not mean a person will be an effective manager. Managers need to know when to activate support services, to recognize symptoms of ill-health in personnel, and also how to proactively manage people working in high-risk occupations (Beyond Blue, 2018; Cook & Mitchell, 2013). Research also supports the benefits of trained PSOs. Individuals who volunteer for a PSO role should undergo a careful selection process, for example being interviewed to enquire about a person's motivation for engaging in the role and their expectations of it. PSOs should be trained in mental health, including understanding their own mental health and self-care. Ongoing professional supervision is essential to maintain the PSOs' mental health and as an ongoing mode of education in assisting and supporting work colleagues in need (Creamer et al., 2012; Scully, 2011; WHO, 2022).

Exemplars of Effective Programs for Frontline Workers

Various programs specific to frontline contexts are discussed in the chapters that follow. Here we mention three programs that have a strong evidence base. The first is a program that has been subjected to comprehensive longitudinal, quantitative, and qualitative research (Tedeschi & Moore, 2019). Warrior PATHH (Progressive and Alternative Training for Helping Heroes) is based on concepts inherent in the PTG model and embodied through the expert companion model (Tedeschi & Calhoun, 2009). Warrior PATHH has been rolled out through the Boulder Crest Foundation in the USA. Boulder Crest was founded by veteran Ken Falke and his wife, Julia, in 2010 (https://bouldercrest.org) and Warrior PATHH commenced in 2014. It is a comprehensive program to promote mental health initially for veterans and their families that later moved to include other types of frontline workers (fire, law enforcement, paramedics). The program starts with a residential retreat of various lengths (e. g., six days) and is integrated with monthly online discussions. The program was redeveloped in consultation with Richard Tedeschi and Brett Moore in 2015 with PTG as its philosophical basis. Tedeschi is the inaugural Chair of the Boulder Crest Institute for Posttraumatic Growth.

As discussed earlier, the need for participatory development of programs that aim to promote mental health, including PTG, is vital to success. Warrior PATHH is facilitated by trained peers. It is a non-clinical program with long-term support, using a growth model to facilitate personal reflections, self-disclosure, and connection with others. It teaches life skills to increase community integration and promote emotional, relational, and spiritual health (https://bouldercrest. org). Longitudinal data attests to the positive impacts of the program. A full report is available at the link provided in the reference list, but in brief, Tedeschi and Moore (2019) cite research that has assessed a large amount of mental health indicators in eight groups who have been through the program, measured at seven time-points across 18 months. Results have demonstrated a 56% reduction in PTSD symptoms, a 57% reduction in anxiety symptoms, 52% less stress, a 39% reduction in sleep disturbances, a 21% increase in self-compassion, and a 58% increase in PTG. These are impressive data, especially given Warrior PATHH is a non-clinical program (i. e., not focused on symptom reduction).

Two other programs aimed at increasing resilience and PTG in frontline personnel were based on an extensive catalogue of work conducted over three decades, led by Shochet and colleagues (e. g., Shochet & Ham, 2004). These programs have been subjected to many Randomized Controlled Trials (e. g., Merry et al., 2004). Adapted from his earlier work, Shochet and colleagues (2011) created another program called the Promoting Resilient Officer (PRO) program which was developed in partnership with a police service. PRO was subjected to a Randomized Control Trial (RCT) with 246 newly recruited police officers who had previously experienced trauma. The new recruits were randomized into psychoeducation as usual or the PRO program which ran as 2-hour workshops each week for seven weeks. Survey data was collected prior to intervention, two months post intervention, and four months after that. There were no group effects on PTSD symptoms but that was probably due to floor effects. In other words, newly recruited police officers go through rigorous psychometric testing prior to being recruited. However, there were significant group differences with increases from T1 to T2 and T1 to T3 in all domains of PTG in the PRO group (Shakespeare-Finch et al., 2014).

Another program for frontline personnel was adapted from PRO to be relevant to mental health nurses, called Promoting Resilience in Nurses (PRiN). Like PRO, PRiN was developed by Shochet and colleagues (Bui et al., 2022) and was also the subject of an RCT. Bui and colleagues (2022) detailed the methods and protocols involved in running the RCT ($n=144$) with mental health nurses, including a waitlist control group during COVID's height and local lockdowns. Embracing the participatory approach, this time the program was run over two full days, three weeks apart. When programs need to suit the organization that they are intended for, the timing of the program often needs to change, for example to accommodate shiftwork. Assessing different programs, inevitably including changes in the timing of delivery, can add to the robustness of evidence for the effectiveness of the program. Data was collected prior to the program, two weeks post program completion and again three months later. Using a nested linear mixed model for each outcome measure, results were very encouraging. Specifically, there were significant increases in coping self-efficacy, wellbeing, and posttraumatic growth between time one and two, and an increase in wellbeing and resilience at time three, controlling for scores on those variables at time one, as well as finding reductions in levels of psychological distress (Foster, 2023).

These programs and their rigorous evaluation lend confidence that psychoeducation and interventions aimed at promoting and fostering mental health in frontline personnel is achievable despite the enormous challenges inherent in such work roles. Indeed, finding significant positive changes in participants who completed the PRiN program, when the RCT was conducted during COVID and lockdowns and considering the enormous pressure on nurses and the entire health system at the time, speaks volumes for the program.

Leadership

Implicit in the above is that a critical element in determining the mental health of frontline personnel is the quality of leadership. For example, poor leadership and a lack of support from supervisors was established as a key factor in the mental ill-health of paramedics (e. g., Harrison, 2019). Trust in leadership has also been related to firefighters' willingness to access support resources when required (Conway & Waring, 2020) and being satisfied with leadership has been related to reductions in burnout in nurses (Zaghini et al., 2020). West and colleagues (2020) wrote an extensive piece detailing ways in which to provide the best possible work context for nurses, thereby improving the quality of care nurses are able to provide their patients. One of the key recommendations was issues pertaining to culture and leadership. They asserted that compassionate leadership and an environment of care and nurturance, which stems from those in leadership positions, is vital for high quality staff support.

Sweeney and colleagues (2022) provide a comprehensive second edition of their 2011 text about leadership in the military, emergency and first responder services. Throughout the chapters, many of which are written by leaders in frontline high-risk occupations, there are some common themes. The first is that good leaders can learn to be good leaders, leveraging their strengths and improving their skills in communication, support, and in mental health so they may more readily identify when a person or group they are leading needs extra assistance. They can learn where to access needed resources at times of need and develop a culture whereby accessing mental health assistance is not met with the common stigma that has dogged frontline personnel accessing assistance for decades. Good leaders are open, they listen, they inspire, and they help to nurture and develop others.

Summary

This chapter has highlighted some of the themes that permeate the chapters in this text. It has highlighted the vital role of evidence-based interventions, psychoeducation, and support, including the vital roles of PSOs and leaders. In the following chapters academics, researchers, clinicians, and frontline personnel provide a glimpse into the worlds of 14 different frontline contexts. The chapters are a mix of international research and practices with application of knowledge gained through research and practice to the various frontline contexts, in order to buffer against the negative impacts of trauma exposure and to promote resilience, PTG, and mental health more broadly. Many of the chapters also include examples of programs not reviewed in this chapter, created at a local level to support a particular staff group.

References

Beyond Blue (2018). Developing a workplace mental health strategy. A how-to guide for organizations. https://www.headsup.org.au/docs/default-source/resources/393615_1117_bl1833_acc-2.pdf

Bui, M. V., McInnes, E., Ennis, G., & Foster, K. (2022). Protocol for a mixed methods process evaluation of the promoting resilience in Nurses (PRiN) trial. *International Journal of Nursing, 31*, 687–696. doi:10.1111/inm.12989

Burchill, C. N. (2019). Critical incident stress debriefing: Helpful, harmful, or neither? *Journal of Emergency Nursing, 45*, 611–612. doi:org/10.1016/j.jen.2019.08.006

Cherry, N., Galarneau, J-M, Haynes, W., Sluggett, B. (2021). The role of organizational supports in mitigating mental ill health in firefighters: a cohort study in Alberta, Canada. *American Journal of Industrial Medicine, 64*, 593–601. doi:10.1002/ajim.23249

Conway, R. R., & Waring, S. (2020). Facilitators and barriers to developing firefighter resilience. *Disaster Prevention and Management, 30*, 327–339. doi:10.1108/DPM-06-2018-0186

Cook, B., & Mitchell, W. (2013). *Occupational health effects for firefighters: The extent and implications of physical and psychological injuries.* Report prepared for the United Firefighters Union of Australia, Victoria Branch. Centre of Full Employment and Equity. https://s3.ap-southeast-2.amazonaws.com/hdp.au.prod.app.vic-engage.files/3914/8609/8798/Attachment_-_UFU_Submission_to_FSR_-_ANNEXURE_59.PDF

Creamer, M., Varker, T., Bisson, J., Darte, K., Greenberg, N., Lau, W., Moreton, G., O'Donnell, M., Richardson, D., Ruzek, J., Watson, P., & Forbes, D. (2012). Guidelines for peer support in high-risk organizations: An international consensus study using the Delphi method. *Journal of Traumatic Stress Studies, 25*, 134–141. doi:10.1002/jts.21685

Feuer, B. S. (2021). First Responder Peer Support: An Evidence-Informed Approach. *Journal of Police and Criminal Psychology, 36,* 365–371. doi:10.1007/s11896-020-09420-z

Foster, K. (2023). *PRiN Randomized Controlled Trial Findings.* Carson Conference Centre,Australian Nursing and Midwifery Federation – Victorian Branch, Melbourne, Australia

Freckelton, I. (2008). *Employers' duties for reasonably foreseeable psychiatric injuries: Hegarty v Queensland Ambulance Service QCA, Psychiatry, Psychology and Law, 15,* 17–24. doi:10.1080/13218710801979092

Harrison, J. (2019). Organisational factors: impacting on health for ambulance personnel. *International Journal of Emergency Services, 8,* 134–146. doi:10.1108/IJES-02-2018-0013

Kim, J., Aggarwal, A., Maloney, S., & Tibbits, M. (2021). Organizational assessment to implement trauma-informed care for first responders, child welfare providers, and healthcare professionals. *Professional Psychology: Research and Practice, 52,* 569–578. doi:10.1037/pro0000408

McDiarmid, M., Condon, M., & Gaitens, J. (2021). The healthcare sector employer's duty of care: Implications for worker wellbeing. *International Journal of Environmental Research and Public Health, 18,* 6015. doi:10.3390/ijerph18116015

Merry, S., McDowell, H., Wild, C., Bir, J., & Cuncliffe, R. (2004). A randomized placebo-controlled trial of a school-based depression prevention program. *Journal of the American Academy of Child & Adolescent Psychiatry, 43,* 538–547. doi: 10.1097/00004583-200405000-00007

Mitchell, J. T., & Everly, G. S., Jr. (1995). Critical incident stress debriefing (CISD) and the prevention of work-related traumatic stress among high-risk occupational groups. In G. S. Everly Jr., & J. M. Laring (Eds.) *Psychotraumatology. The Springer Series on Stress and Coping.* Springer. doi:10.1007/978-1-4899-1034-9_16

Phoenix Australia – Centre for Posttraumatic Mental Health. (2020). *Specific Populations and Trauma Types: Emergency services personnel in Australian Guidelines for the Prevention and Treatment of Acute Stress Disorder, Posttraumatic Stress Disorder and Complex Posttraumatic Stress Disorder.* Melbourne: Phoenix Australia. Retrieved 13 December 2022 from: https://www.phoenixaustralia.org/wp-content/uploads/2022/08/Chapter-9-3.-Emergency-services-personnel-1.pdf

Rose, S., Bisson, J., Churchill, R., & Wesseley, S. (2002). Psychological debriefing for preventing posttraumatic stress disorder (PTSD). *Cochrane Database Systematic Review CD000560.* doi: 10.1002/14651858. CD000560

Scully, P. J. (2011). Taking care of staff: A comprehensive model of support for paramedics and emergency medical dispatchers. *Traumatology, 17,* 35–42. doi:10.1177/1534765611430129

Shakespeare-Finch, J. (2007). Building Resilience in Emergency Service Personnel through Organisational Structures. In Moore, K. (Ed.) *Psychology Making an Impact: Proceedings of the 42nd Conference of the*

Australian Psychological Society. Australian Psychological Society, Australia, pp. 362–365

Shakespeare-Finch, J., Shochet, I., Roos, C., Craig, C., Armstrong, D., Young, R., & Wurfl, A. (2014). *Promoting posttraumatic growth in police recruits: Preliminary results of a randomised controlled resilience intervention trial.* Paper presented to the Australia & New Zealand Disaster & Emergency Management Conference, Surfers Paradise (QLD), 5–7 May

Shakespeare-Finch, J., & Daley, E. (2017). Workplace Belongingness, Psychological Distress and Resilience in Emergency Service Workers. *Psychological Trauma: Research, Theory Practice & Policy, 9,* 32–35. doi:10.1037/tra0000108

Shochet, I., & Ham, D. (2004). Universal School-based Approaches to Preventing Adolescent Depression: Past Findings and Future Directions of the Resourceful Adolescent Program. *International Journal of Mental Health Promotion, 6,* 17–25

Shochet, I. M., Shakespeare-Finch, J., Young, R., Brough, P., Craig, C., Roos. C., Wurfl, A., & Hodge, R. (2011). The development of the Promoting Resilience Officers (PRO) program. *Traumatology, 17,* 43–51

Sweeney. P., Matthews, M. D., Lester, P. D., Sean, H., & Reed, B. (Eds.) (2022). *Leadership in dangerous situations: A handbook for the armed services, emergency services and first responders.* Nava Institute Press

Tedeschi, R. G., & Calhoun, L. G. (2009). The clinician as expert companion. In C. L. Park, S. C. Lechner, M. H. Antoni, & A. L. Stanton (Eds.), *Medical illness and positive life change: Can crisis lead to personal transformation?* (pp. 215–235). American Psychological Association. doi:10.1037/11854-012

Tedeschi, R. G., & Moore, B. (2019). *Warrior PATHH: Final 18-month results. Boulder Crest Institute for Posttraumatic Growth.* https://bouldercrest.org/wp-content/uploads/2022/05/Small_Digital_Vol-4_18-Month-Study.pdf

Tedeschi, R. G., Shakespeare-Finch, J., Taku, K., & Calhoun, L. G. (2018). *Posttraumatic Growth: Theory, Research and Applications.* New York, NY: Routledge

West, M., Bailey, S., & Williams, E. (2020). *The courage of compassion: Supporting nurses and midwives to deliver high-quality care.* https://www.kingsfund.org.uk/sites/default/files/2020-09/The%20courage%20of%20compassion%20full%20report_0.pdf

World Health Organization (2019). *Psychological debriefing in people exposed to a recent traumatic event.* https://www.who.int/mental_health/mhgap/evidence/resource/other_complaints_q5.pdf?ua=1

World Health Organization. (2022). *Guidelines on Mental Health at Work.* Geneva: World Health Organization. License: CC BY-NC-SA 3.0 IGO. Cataloguing-in-Publication (CIP) data. Retrieved 8 December 2022 from: https://www.who.int/publications/i/item/9789240053052

Zaghini, F., Fiorini, J., Piredda, M., Fida, R., & Sili, A. (2020). The relationship between nurse managers' leadership style and patients' perception of the quality of the care provided by nurses: Cross sectional survey. *International Journal of Nursing Studies*, *101*, 103446. doi:10.1016/j.ijnurstu.2019.103446

Specific Frontline Roles and Contexts

part II

Emergency Medical Dispatchers 3

Renée Treloar-Munro

Brayden

Brayden is an EMD in a busy communications centre reflecting on his past three years in the role. He recalls the initial days of adjusting to the role and that it was really difficult moving from an active role as a tradesman to the sedentary role of an EMD where he stands or sits for 12 hours at the same location, and says that he works really hard to stay fit and look after himself when he is away from the work-place. He talks about his role with a lot of positivity and expresses that he is committed to this role as he loves the internal reward of helping people. Brayden reports some frustration with the limits placed on how much help he can provide to callers at times, stating, "We're in the job to care about people and we would like to express that to them, but it is difficult because you can't deviate off of the protocol and help in the way we want to."

Brayden recalls some of his first solo shifts answering emergency calls and receiving a call for a paediatric cardiac arrest. He remembers clearly the sound of a mother screaming and crying as he instructed her on first-aid procedures and noticed that he was picturing the scene of the incident vividly as he listened to the mother frantically administering CPR. After the call, he initially thought he would take a short break, but then noticed how busy the centre was that day and chose to stay and take more emergency phone calls. He was relieved to find the next few calls were very straightforward and he believed that continuing to work after such a "big job" was beneficial to him because it kept him productive and reminded him there are lots of lower acuity calls as part of the job. Sometimes after the big jobs or the jobs that "rattled" his cage, Brayden would notice aspects of the call would keep "popping back into" his head many hours later. He noticed on those days that he needed to run through the call with a colleague to make sure he did everything he was able to do in line with protocols and would often assure himself afterwards saying "you did all you could – it is just how it goes sometimes." After work on those "big job" days, he would unwind from work with physical

DOI: 10.4324/9781003292807-5

exercise, a strict sleeping and eating routine, and giving his family extra hugs and appreciating being with them, and he noticed that he would feel much more tired for a few days afterwards. He said some of the toughest jobs for him were the ones where the media would report on the incident repeatedly and it became harder to switch off from work and get back to his "normal life." He would have to make a concerted effort to turn off the TV after those jobs. Brayden's most rewarding jobs were assisting in the delivery of a baby and said he has had a handful of those really special jobs while he has been in the role.

Emergency Medical Dispatchers (EMDs) are the first point of contact in a medical or psychiatric emergency and support members of the community from the moment they call 000 or 911 for assistance, depending on the country, to the time when paramedics arrive at the scene of the emergency. Despite being an important link in the process of saving lives, the hidden nature of EMD work means that their psychological functioning and their experiences of work and providing emergency support to patients have received far less attention than other emergency roles. Recurrent themes from research paint a clear picture of the EMD role being one with many challenges, including physical and mental health challenges as is highlighted in Brayden's story (Adams, 2012; Smith et al., 2019; Treloar, 2014), as well as a role where there is great potential for posttraumatic growth (PTG) following exposure to trauma (Adams et al., 2015; Ragger et al., 2019; Rees, 2012; Shakespeare-Finch & Adams, 2017; Shakespeare-Finch et al., 2015).

This chapter will review the health of EMDs using a salutogenic approach and will commence by examining the motivations for becoming an EMD, then review the prevalence of stress and psychopathology in EMDs. The role of social support and managerial support for mental health will be discussed, followed by an examination of the research that has examined resilience and PTG in EMDs. The chapter concludes with factors and programs, at the individual and organizational level, that have been found to be associated with the mental health of EMDs.

Motivation to be an EMD

Similar to other health workers, one of the key motivations reported by EMDs for why they chose to apply for the role is their desire to help people (Adams, 2012; Treloar, 2014). Juxtaposed to the motivation of "helping" is the reality of the EMD role which is guided by strict protocols that EMDs are required to adhere to, thus precluding the EMD from connecting with the caller in a more personalized way as highlighted by Brayden's vignette where he states "we're in the job to care about people and we would like to express that to them, but it is difficult because you can't deviate off of the protocol and help in the way we want to." While EMDs may not feel closely connected to most of their callers due to call-taking protocols, the broad theme of knowing they have helped in the process of saving lives is still rewarding to EMDs and particular calls, such as those where they assist in the delivery of a baby over the phone, are particularly memorable and rewarding for EMDs (Adams, 2012; Treloar, 2014).

In order to understand the qualities, life situation, and wellbeing of people who apply to work in the EMD frontline role, Treloar (2014) undertook longitudinal research with a group of newly recruited EMDs which initially revealed this group had significantly higher levels of optimism, resilience, satisfaction with life, and flourishing than the general population. The only factor that continued to be reported as significantly higher than the general population for EMDs after 12 months or more in the role was optimism. Although based on very small numbers, this research also found that any newly recruited EMDs that reported high levels of emotional exhaustion or clinically elevated depression, anxiety, or stress symptoms were unlikely to successfully complete the training associated with this difficult role. That is, out of the 8 EMDs that were experiencing distress symptoms before they commenced in the role, 7 dropped out of the role without completing their first year of training.

Perceived Stress in the Role

Adjustment to the EMD role due to the critical nature of the work and the significant training requirement involved is an area of perceived stress for EMDs. In the vignette, Brayden emphasizes adjusting to the physical health challenges during his first year in the role, as well as to the mental challenges of the role associated with distressing calls. Adams (2012) undertook a significant body of research with EMDs which found that 86% of EMDs discussed the first 1–2 years in the role as being an intense learning curve that created a lot of pressure and feelings of being overwhelmed. Fifty-seven percent of those EMDs also discussed experiencing intrusive thoughts and ruminations and having to learn to adapt to the role by employing new cognitive strategies. Similar to this, Brayden discusses the strategies he uses to cope with stressful calls, which are a mix of emotional, cognitive, and behavioral strategies.

Across 16 different studies, narrative synthesis research by Golding and colleagues (2017) indicated the factors most commonly reported by EMDs to be related to stress are lacking control over high workload, working in under-resourced and pressured environments, and lack of support from management. Shakespeare-Finch and Adams (2017) highlight through lived experience narratives from EMDs the pressure of "Big Brother" (management/quality assurance) watching and questioning their every move in the role. For the dispatching part of the role, allocating paramedic crews to each job when there are not enough crews available can be stressful, with lived experiences from EMDs highlighting that "when a crew is not available when needed, the EMD is questioned as to what they are doing about the workload" (Shakespeare-Finch & Adams, 2017). Another study found that EMDs are given considerably less latitude in the way they perform their role than paramedics, with little downtime to reflect between jobs, and this may restrict an EMD's ability to adapt and increase their resilience in the role (Treloar, 2014).

On a physiological level, research has shown that perceived levels of stress are supported by actual stress hormone levels in the body. Specifically, studies have found that cortisol levels (stress hormone secreted) are higher among EMDs throughout their workday than among gender and age-matched control participants (who were a group of laboratory staff asked not to undertake any physically strenuous work or exercise during the day to obtain reliable daytime, baseline cortisol levels) (Weibel et al., 2003). In Weibel and colleagues' research, there was also a positive correlation between perceived stress reported by EMD participants and the amount of cortisol being secreted. Although research hasn't specifically explored shift-work impacts on cortisol levels (day shifts have only been measured previously), research with EMDs suggests shift-work has an inverse relationship with posttraumatic stress disorder (PTSD) variables, meaning that those who worked a shift-work roster actually reported significantly fewer PTSD symptoms (Shakespeare-Finch et al., 2015). Some research suggests that as well as the work role and organizational factors already mentioned as being related to stress, environmental factors such as poor lighting and loud noise levels are positively correlated with increased stress levels in EMD centers (Smith et al., 2019). Given the impacts of persistent cortisol secretion on health and cognitive function, interventions that target the EMD job setup and environments to reduce stress are crucial. Research has consistently found that factors that are helpful in managing stress for EMDs are peer support and social support from friends and family (Golding et al., 2017, Rees, 2012; Treloar, 2014).

Prevalence of Psychiatric Disorders

Rates of psychopathology among EMDs vary greatly across services and research studies. While some services report rates across all ambulance functions to be as low as .03% for psychological injury (Scully, 2011), others report those rates to be much higher and up to 27% (Petrie et al., 2018). One of the shortfalls of many of the higher-end reports of psychopathology is that it is measured by screening measures, rather than detailed clinical interviews with diagnosed conditions. Another key limitation in the reporting of psychopathology data among EMDs is that, to date, little research has focused on EMDs specifically.

PTSD symptom screening among EMD groups has been conducted in Germany and Australia with rates of PTSD symptoms at clinical levels being reported from 11.3% to 20.5% respectively (Kindermann, 2020; Rees, 2012). Life variables such as a higher number of children and the absence of a secure attachment style were associated with elevated levels of trauma symptomatology (Kindermann et al., 2020). Among EMDs who had experienced traumatic calls, PTSD symptomatology reported indicated that most EMDs rated their PTSD symptoms as manageable in terms of distress. In this research, factors that further predicted lower levels of PTSD symptoms were receiving social support and shift-work (Shakespeare-Finch et al., 2015). The researchers suggest that EMD shift-workers develop strong social connections within their working teams due to their shift patterns, and, in turn, this social support received from their colleagues may buffer the effects of traumatic work on their psychological health.

In another study, for EMDs who had been employed for more than one year in an Australian Centre, one in four respondents reported clinically elevated depression, anxiety, and stress symptoms measured with the Depression, Anxiety, and Stress scale (DASS21). This included 18% who reported clinically elevated anxiety symptoms, 16% with depression symptoms, and 13% with elevated stress symptoms (Treloar, 2014). Research with German EMDs found clinically elevated anxiety symptoms in 7% of respondents, and clinically elevated depression symptoms in 15% of respondents (Kindermann, et al., 2020). Response bias may contribute to some differences between the studies. That is, in the Treloar research 100% participation rates were observed, while in the Kindermann research, there was only a 73% participation rate with one of the main reasons for non-response being they didn't wish to disclose their emotional state (thus potentially leading to underreporting of psychopathology).

Resilience

While early research with EMDs focused on the treatment of psychopathology once a worker became unwell, research over the past two decades has been exploring the predictors of wellbeing and resilience for EMDs in order to reduce the risk of negative health outcomes and foster growth and flourishing in the role (Adams, 2012; Bilsker et al., 2019; Miller et al., 2017; Shakespeare-Finch, 2005; Steinkopf et al., 2018; Treloar, 2014). Psychological resilience in the EMD context looks at the ability of an individual to bounce back from adversity in the role (such as a potentially traumatic call) with short-term emotional distress that does not impede their overall daily functioning significantly (Bonanno, 2005; Miller et al., 2017). Although research has found that resilience levels among EMDs are similar to the general population, studies have also found a number of factors that bolster or diminish resilience levels for this group (Bilsker et al., 2019; Steinkopf et al., 2018).

Steinkopf and colleagues (2018) researched the impact of stress and resilience among EMDs and the impact of these on wellbeing and psychopathology. They found that resilience was negatively correlated with job stress and positively correlated with PTG. Through a series of regression analyses, these researchers also found that for EMDs positive affect was a significant predictor of resilience and that both of these factors taken together significantly predicted PTG. The researchers surmised that resilience was a key protective factor for preventing psychopathology, and that developing resilience involved a willingness to seek help or assistance when stressed. The notion of willingness to seek support to develop resilience is highlighted by our vignette, where whenever Brayden noticed he had been distressed by a job (disruption to functioning), he would seek out support from his colleagues and often feel better following these discussions (return to normal functioning).

Treloar's (2014) research found that on average, EMDs resilience levels are similar to the general population. Among this group, 27% of EMDs reported high levels of resilience, 63% normal levels of resilience and 10% low levels of resilience. Bilsker and colleagues (2019) specifically set out to investigate what factors may be important to bolstering the resilience of paramedics and EMDs. Through exploratory factor analysis, five elements of resilient coping were discovered: balance (life), self-acceptance, trusted social support (colleagues), meaningful work (fulfillment and alignment with values and beliefs), and physical self-care. In support of the importance of meaningful work in resilience development, Miller et al. (2017) also found that resilience was positively associated with compassion satisfaction which measures satisfaction with meaning and purpose in the role. In another study, Shakespeare-Finch et al. (2017) found that workplace belongingness (trusted social support) both reduced distress levels and increased resilience levels. Further research focusing on implementing and testing the effectiveness of programs that target each of these areas would be of benefit to EMDs.

Posttraumatic Growth

Posttraumatic Growth is conceptualized as an emergence of new meaning in life when people who are exposed to extraordinary events, such as trauma, experience positive changes following the event including experiencing changes in relating to others, seeing new possibilities, changes in personal strength, spiritual changes, and a new appreciation for life (Shakespeare-Finch et al., 2003; Tedeschi & Calhoun, 1996). Posttraumatic growth among emergency workers has been found across numerous studies, and the presence of both PTSD symptoms and PTG factors in individuals suggests that positive and negative outcomes from work exposure to trauma can co-exist (Oginska-Bulik, 2015; Ragger et al., 2019; Shakespeare-Finch & Lurie-Beck, 2014). Some quantitative research with EMDs has found PTG and PTSD to be discrete constructs, however, limits around the generalizability of these results are that restricted categories of trauma were analyzed rather than a wide range of traumas (Rees, 2012). Specific to EMDs, qualitative research has painted a clear theme of the interplay of PTG and PTSD symptoms (Adams et al., 2015; Shakespeare-Finch, & Adams, 2017). Rees (2012) reported that almost 80% of EMDs do not experience high levels of distress in response to a traumatic event and found moderate levels of PTG among EMDs. Qualitative research undertaken with EMDs looking at the concept of salutogenesis and growth following trauma suggests that through self-disclosure and self-reflective talk, EMDs can process traumatic events to find positive changes such as improvements in personal strength and having a new appreciation for life (Adams, 2012; Treloar, 2014). In line with the salutogenic model, Brayden also describes a process by which he notices intrusions and ruminations following trauma, and that discussion of this with a colleague aids in his adaptive processing and being able to have a sense of coherence about the event.

EMDs have described their lived experiences in the role with themes of exposure to repeated trauma, followed by intrusions, avoidance, and hyperarousal, and finally themes of PTG and an emergence of new life meaning as they adapt to the role (Adams et al., 2015; Shakespeare-Finch, & Adams, 2017). While at times the protocols in the role can be frustrating to EMDs such as Brayden, it does provide them with a clear boundary to what they may deliver, which potentially assists with their manageability, and thus, a sense of coherence in the role.

When assessing specifically what factors may be at play in promoting PTG among EMDs, receiving social support has been found to be a positive predictor of wellbeing and PTG and a negative predictor of PTSD (Shakespeare-Finch et al., 2015). This research also demonstrated that self-efficacy was a positive predictor of wellbeing. Further research exploring how to promote wellbeing and posttraumatic growth among EMDs is still needed given that early research suggests a different wellbeing profile to other emergency workers, and that experiences of and processing of trauma may different.

Individual Strategies for Coping with the Role

So far, research has suggested that EMDs have higher levels of perceived stress and cortisol levels than the general population and that up to one in four EMDs experience elevated levels of depression, anxiety, stress, or PTSD symptomatology. Research also suggests that EMD wellbeing as measured by resilience, flourishing, and life satisfaction is at similar levels to the general population. So how do EMDs stay healthy and grow in the role? EMDs use a range of adaptive and maladaptive coping strategies with a preference for using a broader range of adaptive strategies to a moderate extent (Treloar, 2014). Adaptive strategies EMDs use include seeking social support, black humor, acceptance, active coping, and reframing (Adams, 2012; Treloar, 2014). Maladaptive strategies of self-blame, substance use, and avoidance behaviors are also utilized by EMDs, but these are to a lesser extent than adaptive strategies (Treloar, 2014). To engage in adaptive coping behaviors, stress and salutogenesis research indicates an individual must have good levels of self-efficacy, that is, their belief in the manageability of the stressor. This is congruent with EMD research which has found self-efficacy to be a crucial factor in promoting EMD wellbeing (Shakespeare-Finch et al., 2015). Research has also found that EMDs who have a secure attachment style may have fewer symptoms of PTSD following exposure to trauma (Kindermann et al., 2020). The likely explanation for this is that those who are securely attached are more likely to have a range of supports in place and will access them when needed. As well as a reduction in PTSD symptoms, EMDs who also actively utilize their social supports to cope with aspects of the role are also experiencing benefits to wellbeing and PTG (Shakespeare-Finch et al., 2015). Social supports used by EMDs include family (95%), friends (80%), work colleagues (45%), and specially trained peer support officers (18%; Rees, 2012).

Organizational Approach to Coping with the Role

There have been relatively few organizational level interventions undertaken and analyzed in support of assisting with the coping of EMDs in the role across the world. Some recent research to investigate the viability of the mobile application "PTSD Coach" to reduce PTSD symptoms revealed some benefits of using the application for one month (Willis, 2019). Importantly, the study found a reduction in alcohol use as well as a reduction in depression, anxiety, anger, and PTSD symptoms. The program was only moderately helpful in encouraging people to seek social support and discuss difficult cases which we know are important components of PTG.

Beyond Blue (2016, 2018) has published a range of recommendations for first responder organizations to assist with supporting all first responders from recruitment through to retirement. The strategies put in place are to reduce the level of risk associated with the potentially traumatic work of EMDs. A program developed for paramedics and EMDs specifically within an Australian ambulance organization encapsulates all components recommended by Beyond Blue (Scully, 2011; Shakespeare-Finch et al., 2014). This program has been in place for 30 years and has been reviewed and refined periodically. It includes mental health preparedness training with all new EMDs with a focus on PTSD symptoms and salutogenesis; individualized reflective work and counseling support for the development of coping skills while adjusting to the role; the ongoing availability of counselors throughout their career which can be accessed for any work or personal reason; and proactive and reactive peer support officer (PSO) contact for critical and potentially traumatic incidents, as well as supervisor mental health training. In the most recent review of the program, EMDs reported a desire to have more PSOs and counselors with greater job-specific knowledge of the EMD role specifically (Shakespeare-Finch et al., 2014). EMDs also requested greater levels of connection and contact within their organization and more information and support for mental health and wellbeing. From what is known about other EMD organizations around the world, there are relatively few with any sort of staff support system in place. Based on available EMD research, any programs which bolster self-efficacy, social supports, and belongingness will have positive health impacts for EMDs.

Conclusion

Aspects of the EMD role and environment can impact the physical and emotional wellbeing of people who perform that role. This chapter has highlighted that of greatest consideration for workplaces is the need to understand the intricacies of the EMD role and how it is different in many ways from other emergency response roles, and to provide appropriate proactive training and support for EMDs to keep them physically and emotionally strong in the role. This chapter highlighted that perceptions of stress are high among this group and that interventions for reducing stress levels are required, including review of the amount of calls being managed within a work shift to facilitate opportunities for adaptive processing and growth, and building stronger managerial relationships. In line with a salutogenic approach to processing trauma, this chapter has demonstrated that while PTSD symptoms are reported among some EMDs, other EMDs report PTG in the role, particularly where self-efficacy, social support, and sense of belongingness are high. A thorough and considered approach to supporting staff within the EMD environment is required, with a focus on proactive and reactive strategies for maintaining the wellbeing of these people and with an emphasis on the factors that have been shown to benefit this group specifically.

References

Adams, K. (2012). *The lived experiences of emergency medical dispatchers: An interpretative phenomenological analysis*. Honors thesis, Queensland University of Technology. Queensland

Adams, K., Shakespeare-Finch, J., & Armstrong, D. (2015). Interpretative Phenomenological Analysis of stress and well-being in Emergency Medical Dispatchers. *Journal of Loss and Trauma, 20,* 430–448. doi:10.1080/15325024.2014.949141

Bilsker, D., Gilbert, M., Alden, L., Sochting, I., & Khalis, A. (2019). Basic dimensions of resilient coping in paramedics and dispatchers. *Australasian Journal of Paramedicine, 16.* doi:10.33151/ajp.16.690

Beyond Blue (2016). *Good practice framework for mental health and wellbeing in first responder organisations.* www.beyondblue.org.au

Beyond Blue (2018). *Answering the Call. National Survey on Police and Emergency Services.* www.beyondblue.org.au

Bonanno, G. (2005) Resilience in the face of trauma. *Current Directions in Psychological Science, 14,* 135–138. doi:10.1111/j.0963-7214.2005.00347.x

Golding S. E., Horsfield, C., Davies, A., Egan, B., Jones, M., Raleigh, M., Schofield, P.,

Kindermann, D., Sanzenbacher, M., Nagy, E., Greinacher, A., Cranz, A., Nikendei, A., Friederich, H. C., & Nikendei, C. (2020). Prevalence and risk factors of secondary traumatic stress in emergency call-takers and dispatchers - a cross-sectional study. *European Journal of Psychotraumatology, 11*(1), 1799478. doi:10.1080/20008198.2020.1799478

Miller, A., Unruh, L., Zhang, N., Liu, X., & Wharton, T. (2017). Professional quality of life of Florida emergency medical dispatchers. *International Journal of Emergency Services, 6*(1), 29–39. https://www.emerald.com/insight/content/doi/10.1108/IJES-01-2017-0001/full/html

Oginska-Bulik, N. (2015). Social support and negative and positive outcomes of experienced traumatic events in a group of male emergency service workers. *International Journal of Occupational Safety and Ergonomics (JOSE), 21*(2), 119–127. doi:10.1080/10803548.2015.1028232

Petrie, K., Milligan-Saville, J., Gayed, A., Deady, M., Phelps, A., Dell, L., Forbes, D., Bryant, R. A., Calvo, R. A., Glozier, N., & Harvey, S. B. (2018). Prevalence of PTSD and common mental disorders amongst ambulance personnel: a systematic review and meta-analysis. *Social Psychiatry & Psychiatric Epidemiology, 53,* 897–909. doi:10.1007/s00127-018-1539-5

Ragger, K., Hiebler-Ragger, M., Herzog, G., Kapfhammer, H. P., & Unterrainer, H. F. (2019). Sense of coherence is linked to post-traumatic growth after critical incidents in Austrian ambulance personnel. *BMC* Psychiatry, *19,* 89. doi:10.1186/s12888-019-2065-z

Rees, A. (2012). *Emergency medical dispatchers: Impacts of self-efficacy and social support on well-being and post-trauma responses.* Bachelor of Behavioural Science (Honours) Psychology, School of Psychology and Couselling, Queensland University of Technology

Scully, P. J. (2011). Taking care of staff: A comprehensive model of support for paramedics and emergency medical dispatchers. *Traumatology, 17,* 35–42. doi:10.1177/1534765611430129.

Shakespeare-Finch, J., & Adams, K. (2017) Growth and meaning from negotiating the complex journey of being an Emergency Medical Dispatcher. In E. Altmaier (Ed). *Reconstructing Meaning after Trauma* (pp. 117–132). London, UK: Elsevier

Shakespeare-Finch, J., & Lurie-Beck, J. (2014). A meta-analytic clarification of the relationship between posttraumatic growth and symptoms of posttraumatic distress disorder. *Journal of Anxiety Disorders, 28*(2), 223–229.doi: 10.1016/j.janxdis.2013.10.005

Shakespeare-Finch, J., Wehr, T., Kaiplinger, I., & Daley, E. (2014). *Caring for emergency service personnel. Does what we do work?* Australia & New Zealand Disaster & Emergency Management Conference, Surfers Paradise (QLD), 5th–7th May. https://eprints.qut.edu.au/73083/21/ANZDEM.QAS.pdf

Shakespeare-Finch, J., Rees, A., & Armstrong, D. (2015). Social Support, Self-efficacy,Trauma and Well-Being in Emergency Medical Dispatchers. *Social Indicators Research, 123*, 549–565. doi:10.1007/s11205-014-0749-9

Smith, E. C., Holmes, L., & Burkle, F. M. (2019). Exploring the Physical and Mental Health Challenges Associated with Emergency Service Call-Taking and Dispatching: A Review of the Literature. *Prehospital Disaster Medicine, 34*, 619–624. doi:10.1017/S1049023X19004990

Squires, A., Start, K., Quinn, T., & Cropley, M. (2017). Exploring the psychological health of emergency dispatch centre operatives: a systematic review and narrative synthesis. *PeerJ 5:e3735*. doi:10.7717/peerj.3735

Steinkopf, B., Reddin, R., Black, R., Van Hasselt, V., & Couwels, J. (2018). Assessment of stress and resiliency in Emergency Dispatchers. *Journal of Police and Criminal Psychology, 33*, 398–411. doi:10.1007/s11896-018-9255-3

Treloar, R. (2014). *The experiences of Emergency Medical Dispatchers: A qualitative and quantitative evaluation of functioning.* Professional Doctorate, School of Psychology, The University of Queensland. doi:10.14264/341647

Weibel, L., Gabrion, I., Aussedat, M., & Kreutz, G. (2003). Work-related stress in an emergency medical dispatch center. *Emergency Medical Services, 41*(4), 500–506. doi:10.1067/mem.2003.109

Willis, E. (2019). *The Examination of a Mobile Application for the Reduction of Posttraumatic Stress Related Symptoms in Emergency Dispatchers.* Electronic Theses and Dissertations. 6351. Accessed at https://stars.library.ucf.edu/etd/6351

Law Enforcement

4

K.C. Kalmbach

Jake

Jake wakes nearly every day at 3:10am. He jerks awake to the scent and the image of his partner, only two months on the job, lying in a pool of her own blood. The weapon, he remembers distinctly, a Glock, blurry in his peripheral vision. He had looked away, just for a second he told the Sergeant, just for a second, when he heard the crying toddler enter the room. Just for a second, they both turned to look at the shivering, diaper-clad child. That's when he fired – the desperate, hallucinating teenage father. Jake remembers the look on his partner's face, everything in slow motion, eyes widening with shock, as she fell to the trash-littered floor. Jake swung around. He doesn't remember pulling out his gun or making the decision to. Everything goes silent, like someone turned the sound off. But he can see the teenager, knees buckling, propelled forwards, slamming into the filthy floor, his face coming to rest just a few inches from hers. Jake's body-cam records the entire incident – just 006.03.01 seconds in duration. But it's the smell, the scent of propellant and lead dust, that wakes him to stagger to the bathroom and vomit, every morning. It's been 182 days. Used to be he couldn't imagine doing anything else with his life for the next 30 years. Just like his father, and his father's father. Loved listening to all the war stories the old timers would tell, spinning them out, down at the Rusty Nail. How they loved the life; the job. How proud they were. Now, the years stretch out in front of him, like a life sentence. He tries not to think about it. Maybe no one has noticed yet; his GPS will show a clear avoidance of that block despite it being on his beat. Every morning he throws back a few anti-nausea pills with the coffee. A couple more with the Zoloft. Just to get him through the morning shift. They've kept him off graveyard. He didn't ask. No one says anything. One day at a time, he tells himself. Anyone can do one day.

(Identifiers changed; used with permission.)

In 2019, with much fanfare, the U.S. Senate passed a resolution designating October 28th as *National First Responders Day* (U.S. Senate, Committee on

DOI: 10.4324/9781003292807-6

Homeland Security and Governmental Affairs, 2019). Long in the making and bipartisan in nature, it was conceived in response to the murder of Sean Collier, the young Massachusetts Institute of Technology (MIT) police officer who was ambushed by the Boston Marathon bombers. In the U.S., as in other developed nations, first responders have long enjoyed widespread goodwill and public support. And yet, within this group (comprising law enforcement, fire, disaster, and emergency medical/paramedics), a significant divide is opening. A recent poll of Americans showed that a clear majority of those surveyed judged firefighters (80%) and paramedics (76%) to be "trustworthy." However, the percentage who considered law enforcement/police to be trustworthy dipped to only half of those surveyed (49%), and 21% declared police to be "untrustworthy" as a group (IPSOS, 2021).

The corrosive effect of over a decade of U.S. partisan politics is now taking a toll on public trust in one of the most critical and front-facing of public servant professions. Adding stress to an already overburdened system, law enforcement officials report an unprecedented number of people leaving the profession in the past few years; resignations are estimated to be up 20% and retirements 45% (Police Executive Research Forum, 2021). Given that the majority of police departments in the US are small and mid-sized, this exodus is having a significant impact on the communities they serve (Westervelt, 2021). For a job that is already one of the most stressful and risk-laden occupations in civil society, the loss of sworn members as well as public trust is concerning. Potential recruits might understandably wonder if the career is worth pursuing.

Background

For members of the law enforcement community, exposure to potentially traumatic experiences is part of the job description and, indeed, may attract a self-selected segment of the population, who, at a minimum, are not dissuaded by such danger (Burke & Shakespeare-Finch, 2011; Paton, 2005). Historically, much of the research and intervention in this area relied upon three presumptions: (a) law enforcement members experience on-the-job trauma similarly; (b) trauma exposure leads to only negative health outcomes; and (c) leadership and/or organizational factors are, at best, peripheral to the experience of trauma and its sequelae. These presumptions are flawed.

While the prevalence of serious mental health concerns is undeniably elevated in law enforcement populations compared to civilians, it is by no means the only story to be told. In fact, research suggests posttraumatic growth (PTG) and resiliency may be as ubiquitous (Tedeschi et al., 2015). Research has long established the covariance of posttraumatic stress disorder (PTSD) and PTG; in some cases, a positive linear relationship, in others, an inverted-U relationship (Shakespeare-Finch & Lurie-Beck,

2014). Although beyond the scope of this chapter, the expansion of PTSD criterion A in the Diagnostic and Statistical Manual of Mental Disorders, Fifth edition (DSM-5), to include *indirect* exposure complicated the issue by perhaps lowering the threshold for diagnosis, increasing the number of people who qualified and thus obscuring otherwise apparent effects (American Psychiatric Association, 2013). Additionally, some complain of conceptual "bracket creep" and the over-pathologizing of normative responses to stressors, thus potentially undermining adaptive resiliency and further muddying the literature (McNally, 2010). These points are raised to illustrate the fact that there has long been controversy over the issue of "who qualifies" and what trauma "looks like." Acknowledging this operational definition dilemma is critical to understanding why the extant research may, at times, be inconsistent or equivocal. More recently, however, the focus has shifted to the role of individual differences in personality, prior trauma exposure, cognitive schemas (or mental models), adaptive processing, and how positive outcomes may be shaped through intentional and targeted training and intervention.

Under the lens of the salutogenic model, then, some interesting questions pertaining to law enforcement arise: Can cognitive schemas about the world be modified or made flexibly adaptive through intervention (Shochet et al., 2011)? Can an individual be trained or "primed" to respond in a new adaptive manner when confronted with novel traumatic stressors (Dunning, 2003; Linley & Joseph, 2004; Paton & Burke, 2007)? Can PTSD and PTG coexist conceptually and meaningfully within an individual (Chopko, 2010; Horswill et al., 2021; Shakespeare-Finch & Lurie-Beck, 2014)? Does personality interact with trauma to produce differential outcomes (Burke et al., 2006; Burke & Shakespeare-Finch, 2011; Horswill et al., 2021; Kunst et al., 2017; McCanlies et al., 2014)? Can prior exposure (Burke et al., 2006) or organizational factors moderate outcomes (Boothroyd et al., 2019; Horswill et al., 2021; Huddleston et al., 2006; Paton, 2005; Pole et al., 2006; Snell et al., 2014)? Research would suggest the answer is yes, to all the questions posed.

In Jake's case, Jake came to his career by the same path that many military members and first responders do – a family tradition and legacy. It is possible that personality characteristics predisposing him to this career may be both learned and inherited (e.g., impulsivity, risk-taking, altruism, empathy, optimism). To the extent that he is cognitively flexible and possesses innate resilience, it will serve him well. However, if he is high on the neurotic axis or prone to emotion-focused coping, he may struggle. As a member of a multigenerational first responder family, he is likely to have been well aware of the risks as well as rewards of such a choice. Many law enforcement members derive satisfaction and purpose from the experiences that civilians might find aversive. He likely grew up hearing stories about the bizarre and unpredictable ways in which a day can quickly go "sideways" on the job. Positive outcomes will depend upon the extent that Jake can make meaning of the tragedy and process his guilt, shame, and grief, while receiving support from his department (supervisor), family, and friends.

Traumatic Exposure and Health Outcomes

Despite the fact the field continues to be plagued by a lack of measurement standardization, as well as a failure to take demographic variables into account (i.e., most law enforcement members in Western countries are white males, a group prone to high-risk behaviors and adverse outcomes), there is clear evidence that members of law enforcement face higher rates of general stress-related health problems relative to the community.

Suicide and foreshortened lifespans are significant risks for law enforcement (Chopko et al., 2014; Dixon, 2021; Heyman et al., 2018). Drawing on Centers for Disease Control and Prevention (CDC) data from 4.5 million adult decedents from 26 U.S. states, a recent proportionate mortality ratio (PMR) analysis found that law enforcement members (across all job categories) were 54% more likely to die from suicide than the average worker (Violanti & Steege, 2020). In fact, there is some evidence that first responders may be more likely to die by suicide than in the line of duty (Heyman et al., 2018). Another study found that members of the Buffalo, New York law enforcement community died significantly earlier (from all causes) by more than two decades (21.9 years) when compared to U.S. males in general; differences were most marked in the younger age ranges (Violanti et al., 2013).

Equally concerning are the "walking wounded." That is to say, estimates of PTSD in law enforcement populations are in the range of 15–35% (10% in the "severe" range) (Austin-Ketch et al., 2012). Also elevated are insomnia, anxiety, depression (as much as 12%) (Hartley et al., 2011b; Wang et al., 2010), alcohol abuse (Ballenger et al., 2011), and suicidal ideation (up to 8.8%) (Chopko et al., 2014). Conversely, prior exposure to (manageable) trauma (Burke & Shakespeare-Finch, 2011) might promote resiliency and adaptiveness, while self-efficacy (Snell et al., 2014), satisfaction with life, and gratitude (McCanlies et al., 2014) appear to mitigate risk. However, some studies have found that repeated chronic exposure to trauma does not fortify nor enhance resilience but serves rather as a "domino effect," chipping away at self-esteem and a sense of purpose (McCormack & Riley, 2016). Others have found no beneficial impact of enhanced spirituality on distress but rather a positive association, although alcohol use was negatively correlated (Chopko et al., 2016).

Although the foregoing may paint a somewhat disturbing and bleak picture, it is nonetheless important to recognize the incredible amount of hardiness or resiliency those same numbers imply – two-thirds to three-quarters of law enforcement do *not* develop trauma or stressor-related disorders despite facing the same adversity and distressing events.

However, it is important to note the role that inherited traits and epigenetics play in the vulnerability of members to stress-related disorders (Mehta et al., 2022). It is imperative not to make the mistake of conflating symptoms with "strength," or lack thereof, as is often done in stigmatizing narratives about mental illness in law enforcement populations.

In addition to mental health problems, numerous studies have found a higher prevalence of serious health conditions such as obesity, metabolic syndrome, and higher cholesterol levels in law enforcement samples (Hartley et al., 2011a; Hartley et al., 2011b). In terms of prior exposure, 20–25% of U.S. law enforcement report prior military service, an occupation that also carries the risk of trauma exposure and both mental and physical injury (Schafer et al., 2015). Social impacts can be more difficult to assess accurately, and reports of higher rates of divorce, child abuse, and intimate partner violence are hotly contested. Nonetheless, it is safe to presume, given the foregoing, that the private and social lives of law enforcement workers may also manifest the stress that results from the work they do (Mennicke & Ropes, 2016; Woody, 2006). Finally, stigma (both self- and other-focused) may be the greatest preventable danger; numerous studies continue to depict a pervasive culture of silence, shame, and secrecy surrounding traumatic stress and resultant distress in law enforcement and other first responder communities (Karaffa & Koch, 2016).

Although early in his career, Jake would do well to cultivate a healthy lifestyle, incorporating physical, mental, social, and emotional practices which promote wellbeing and connectedness. Jake may have noticed his father or grandfather (and colleagues) engaging in denial or non-productive coping (e.g., drinking, avoidance). Jake has received a Zoloft prescription and hopefully therapy accompanies that medication regime. If he relies solely on prescription pills to avoid the painful and difficult process of therapy, he may be at risk for future substance use problems. He is exhibiting behavioral avoidance and, it seems, emotional and social avoidance. Being of a younger generation, Jake may have learned about mental disorders and the importance of positive affectivity; he may be better informed and carry less stigma about reaching out for assistance. However, departmental culture will likely be the greatest influence on his trajectory. The fact that no one has talked to him about the traumatic event is not promising and suggests a culture of stigma and silence. Avoiding burnout will require proactive measures and if such efforts are supported and promoted by his department and leadership, he will be better equipped to deal with the next traumatic event that confronts him. Without their support, he may flounder.

Posttraumatic Di/Stress and Posttraumatic Growth

Compared to the corpus of research on negative outcomes associated with trauma, investigation of positive outcomes, specifically transformational posttraumatic growth in law enforcement populations, is relatively nascent. Nonetheless, a growing number of rigorous and well-constructed studies from around the globe have found support for the proposition that traumatic stress (variously termed PTSD, PTS, or traumatic distress) is not incompatible with, and, in fact, is often positively correlated with PTG in law enforcement populations (Chopko, 2010; Chopko et al., 2018, 2019; Leppma et al., 2018), or demonstrates an inverted U shaped relationship (Shakespeare-Finch & Lurie-Beck, 2014), similar to other high risk/high trauma groups such as military members and combat veterans (Moore et al., 2020; Tedeschi et al., 2015; Tedeschi & McNally, 2011). Not only do these two constructs coexist, in fact, PTG *requires* a traumatic stressor significant enough to rupture one's existing worldview in order to seed a change so great as to be personally transformative (Tedeschi & Calhoun, 2004).

The association found between PTG and traumatic stress raises the urgent question of how such personally transformative and beneficial effects might be fostered and supported within a field not known for promoting health and wellness within its ranks. Specifically, how might we foster conditions conducive to PTG while acknowledging the very real importance and mission of those tasked with upholding law and order in an oft-times disorderly society? The answer lies within a comprehensive program that embraces both operational and mental health training and intervention. The orienting "north star" of such an approach must explicitly be mission-serving to win leadership buy-in. In other words, such a program must be in the furtherance of (i) public safety and (ii) officer safety. There is no question that any initiative which improves the health and wellness of its members is serving both goals simultaneously. Healthy, functional members can make sound judgments and execute critical calls without endangering themselves, the department, or the public.

Priming for Adaptive Growth in Law Enforcement Members

So, what are the core features of an effective "PTG priming program" for law enforcement? Three pillars are proposed as fundamental elements: (1) organizational support and facilitation; (2) operational training for adaptive capacity; and (3) psychoeducation, intervention, and support.

An incident is only "critical" or "traumatic" when it is interpreted as such by the individual. Events can be experienced, processed, and made sense of in highly idiosyncratic and temporally variable ways. In other words, a critical event occurs when an individual perceives it to fall outside of expected parameters or fails to fit within established mental models or cognitive schemas (of how such things should work or go) (Janoff-Bulman, 1989; Paton & Burke, 2007; Tedeschi & Calhoun, 2004).

Every individual has a highly personalized set of mental models, built up over time and infused with personal experiences, values, and beliefs about themselves, others, and the world writ large. This suggests an important point of leverage for training purposes; by introducing new information or strategies for handling traumatic events, we foster adaptive change and a reconstruction of mental models, expanding a sense of competence and efficacy. Training was able to increase adaptive capacity to new and novel stressors encountered in disaster responders. Prior exposure and familiarity with scenarios became incorporated into new and more flexible cognitive schemas, giving members a sense of competency and allowing them to make meaning out of a broader range of novel and otherwise insensible traumatic events.

Key Recommendations

The first recommendation is given priority because success will be unlikely without committed and consistent buy-in by leadership. Additionally, with law enforcement members, as with military members, it is critical that professionals delivering training and intervention be highly familiar with law enforcement culture (preferably "one of' them"). More so than in other fields (i.e., less high-risk/high-trauma professions), law enforcement members are likely to intuitively trust and find more credible those who have walked in their metaphorical shoes. Equally important is training and experience in the PTG model and "expert companion" orientation (Joseph et al., 2015; Tedeschi et al., 2015), as well as familiarity with current research trends in law enforcement members and the larger first responder community.

Organizational Support and Facilitation

Organizations play a critical role in establishing context and expectations, as well as promoting wellbeing of their members (Paton, 2005). Research is now accumulating which reiterates organizational variables such as "hassles" (i.e., "red tape," lack of consultation, poor communication) and "uplifts" (i.e., feeling empowered, given responsibility, acknowledged for good work) are more powerful predictors of outcomes (i.e., subjective and objective wellbeing, traumatic stress, mental health and wellness) than traumatic incidents themselves (e. g., Huddleston et al., 2006). Law enforcement leadership must appreciate the impact that seemingly minor, day-to-day "hassles" can have on members. Such seemingly trivial variables have the ability to layer on to produce cynicism, burnout, disengagement, poor performance, or even traumatic stress. Leadership must take responsibility for setting the tone and shaping an "organizational climate of care" (Paton, 2005), promulgating procedures and policy to promote engagement, resiliency, restoration, and growth (Boothroyd et al., 2019; Shochet et al., 2011). For trust to be established, law enforcement members will need to see a commitment to ongoing support and funding for such an initiative over the long term.

Operational Training for Adaptive Capacity

Perceptions of uncontrollability and unpredictability are amongst the most destabilizing psychological states for most humans, especially for those tasked with protection and defense. The goal of operational training is to increase the range of situations with which one becomes familiar, thus reducing the sense of vulnerability and enhancing a sense of control (Paton, 2006). To this end, opportunities for training should range from traditional in-class lectures to ride-alongs with other departments or agencies, video, and live-action participation with allied fields (e.g., EMS, fire). This latter option can be helpful because the law enforcement member is not expected to take a leading role and can instead provide support while watching and learning from other first responders. The most effective method may be simulations and live drills. The overarching goal is to expose the member (safely and from a distance) to a wider range of potentially traumatic events so as to broaden and build resilience and capacity. As members witness events that fall outside of their mental models (and which would typically cause distress), they are provided supportive instruction on what to notice, and how to respond, to effectively execute their duties. This type of pre-viewing of potential trauma serves not so much as inoculation as "priming" for future performance (Paton & Burke, 2007).

Psychoeducation, Intervention, and Support

Psychoeducation should take the form of interesting audio/visual content and interactional training which can include role play, topical guest speakers, and "lived experience" peers (e.g., an officer who has experience with PTSD or suicide). Normalization of stress responses should be a priority, and members can be educated in the biopsychosocial model to further help integrate their understanding of how trauma impacts individuals on many levels. Additionally, members should be educated about the benefits reaped from enhancing positivity (Harnett et al., 2021), fostering resiliency by maintaining social connectedness (Pole et al., 2006), and refraining from distancing or avoidant coping.

One exciting finding in the research is the role that prior trauma can play in fostering PTG and building adaptive capacity for subsequent trauma (Burke et al., 2006; Burke & Shakespeare-Finch, 2011). In a similar vein, PTG has been found to be associated with higher levels of adverse childhood events, suggesting that prior (manageable) exposure may serve a positive capacity-building purpose (Horswill et al., 2021). This research can be shared to demonstrate both the ubiquitous experience of trauma (both in and out of service) and how "negative" events can produce positive outcomes depending upon how a person chooses to view, process, and interpret events. Approaching trauma from this angle allows members to see the possibility of proactive reframing or making something useful out of an otherwise aversive experience. Care must be taken to never suggest that trauma is inherently a "good" or "positive" or desirable experience, but rather that what determines the outcome may be a willingness to shift perspectives and do the difficult work of processing traumatic events.

Following psychoeducation efforts, appropriately timed and delivered intervention initiatives can address those who may volunteer or be identified as likely to benefit from one-on-one interaction. Finally, ongoing support should be available in the form of an employee assistance program or other easily accessible and confidential helpline or telehealth option. Examples of a few (highly specialized) successful programs are beginning to reach mainstream awareness (Boothroyd et al., 2019; Joseph et al., 2015; Pole et al., 2006; Shochet et al., 2011; Tedeschi et al., 2015).

Summary

On May 24, 2022, an 18-year-old gunman armed with an automatic rifle entered an elementary school in Uvalde, Texas. Over the course of an hour, unimpeded, he shot dead 19 children and two teachers. Audio from dispatch on that day picked up one girl's whispered plea: "Please send help… I don't wanna die" (Prokupecz et al., 2022).

Modern policing has been thrust forward into a new era by a global pandemic and the unprecedented political, economic, and sociocultural events of the past few years. For the field to remain relevant and thrive, it must adapt and grow. In a similar vein, it is proposed that law enforcement of the future must be prepared and equipped to face dangers and threats previously unknown. Tomorrow's force will need to flexibly adapt and respond to events of a scale and magnitude previously unimagined. To be effective, they must move towards more sophisticated training models and programs that acknowledge and prepare for the inevitable trauma that will be encountered, but also foster characteristics and conditions which lead to posttraumatic adaptation and growth.

In the end, 376 officers, including local, state, and federal agencies, would respond to the scene in Uvalde. Video would reveal chaos, confusion, and fear in the faces of men trained to protect and serve. The words of one 10-year-old child, huddled under a desk and surrounded by the bodies of her classmates, would play out on endless news loops for the next several months:

> "I understand what to do in these situations. My dad taught me when I was a little girl. Send help."

> (Prokupecz et al., 2022)

References

American Psychiatric Association. (2013). *Diagnostic and statistical manual of mental disorders.* (5th ed.). American Psychiatric Association

Austin-Ketch, T., Violanti, J., Fekedulegn, D., Andrew, M. E., Burchfield, C. M., & Hartley, T. A. (2012). Addictions and the Criminal Justice System, What Happens on the Other Side? Post-traumatic Stress Symptoms and Cortisol Measures in a Police Cohort. *Journal of Addictions Nursing, 23,* 22–29. doi:10.3109/10884602.2011.645255

Ballenger, J. F., Best, S. R., Metzler, T. J., Wasserman, D. A., Mohr, D. C., Liberman, A., Delucchi, K., Weiss, D. S., Fagan, J. A., Waldrop, A. E., & Marmar, C. R. (2011). Patterns and Predictors of Alcohol Use in Male and Female Urban Police Officers: Alcohol Use among Urban Police Officers: *The American Journal on Addictions, 20,* 21–29. doi:10.1111/j.1521-0391.2010.00092.x

Boothroyd, R. A., Green, S., & Dougherty, A. (2019). Evaluation of Operation Restore: A brief intervention for first responders exposed to traumatic events. *Traumatology, 25,* 162–171. doi:10.1037/trm0000168

Burke, K. J., & Shakespeare-Finch, J. (2011). Markers of resilience in new police officers: Appraisal of potentially traumatizing events. *Traumatology, 17,* 52–60 doi:10.1177/1534765611430725

Burke, K. J., Shakespeare-Finch, J., Paton, D., & Ryan, M. (2006). Characterizing the resilient officer: Individual attributes at point of entry to policing. *Traumatology, 12*(3), 178–188. doi:10.1177/1534765606296531

Chopko, B. A. (2010). Posttraumatic distress and growth: An empirical study of police officers. *American Journal of Psychotherapy, 64,* 55–72. doi:10.1176/appi.psychotherapy.2010.64.1.55

Chopko, B. A., Facemire, V. C., Palmieri, P. A., & Schwartz, R. C. (2016). Spirituality and health outcomes among police officers: Empirical evidence supporting a paradigm shift. *Criminal Justice Studies: A Critical Journal of Crime, Law & Society, 29,* 363–377. doi:10.1080/1478601X.2016.1216412

Chopko, B. A., Palmieri, P. A., & Adams, R. E. (2018). Relationships among traumatic experiences, PTSD, and posttraumatic growth for police officers: A path analysis. *Psychological Trauma: Theory, Research, Practice, and Policy, 10,* 183–189. doi:10.1037/tra0000261

Chopko, B. A., Palmieri, P. A., & Adams, R. E. (2019). Posttraumatic growth in relation to the frequency and severity of traumatic experiences among police officers in small to midsize departments. *Journal of Interpersonal Violence, 34,* 1247–1260. doi:10.1177/0886260516651089

Chopko, B. A., Palmieri, P. A., & Facemire, V. C. (2014). Prevalence and predictors of suicidal ideation among US law enforcement officers. *Journal of Police and Criminal Psychology, 29,* 1–9. doi:10.1007/s11896-013-9116-z

Dixon, S. S. (2021). Law enforcement suicide: The depth of the problem and best practices for suicide prevention strategies. *Aggression and Violent Behavior, 61.* doi:10.1016/j.avb.2021.101649

Dunning, C. (2003). Sense of coherence in managing trauma workers. In D. Paton, J. M. Violanti, & L. M. Smith (Eds.), *Promoting capabilities to manage posttraumatic stress: Perspectives on resilience* (2003-02891-009; pp. 119–135). Charles C Thomas Publisher, Ltd.; APA PsycInfo https://tamusa.idm.oclc.org/login?url=https://search.ebscohost.com/login.aspx?direct=true&db=psyh&AN=2003-02891-009&site=ehost-live&scope=site

Harnett, P. H., Kelly, M. C., & Gullo, M. J. (2021). The impact of posttraumatic stress disorder on the psychological distress, positivity, and well-being of Australian police officers. *Psychological Trauma: Theory, Research, Practice, and Policy, 15,* 340–348. doi:10.1037/tra0001136

Hartley, T. A., Burchfiel, C. M., Fekedulegn, D., Andrew, M. E., Knox, S. S., & Violanti, J. M. (2011a). Associations between police officer stress and the metabolic syndrome. *International Journal of Emergency Mental Health, 13,* 243–256. APA PsycInfo

Hartley, T. A., Burchfiel, C. M., Fekedulegn, D., Andrew, M. E., & Violanti, J. M. (2011b). Health disparities in police officers: Comparisons to the US general population. *International Journal of Emergency Mental Health, 13,* 211–220. APA PsycInfo

Heyman, M., Dill, J., & Douglas, R. (2018). *The Ruderman White Paper on mental health and suicide of first responders.* https://www.firefightermentalhealth.org/system/files/First%20Responder%20White%20Paper_Final.pdf

Horswill, S. C., Jones, N. A., & Carleton, R. N. (2021). Psychosocial factors associated with Canadian police officers' susceptibility to posttraumatic stress and growth. *Canadian Journal of Behavioural Science / Revue Canadienne Des Sciences Du Comportement, 53,* 285–295. doi:10.1037/cbs0000221

Huddleston, L. M., Paton, D., & Stephens, C. (2006). Conceptualizing traumatic stress in police officers: Preemployment, critical incident, and organizational influences. *Traumatology, 12,* 170–177. doi:10.1177/1534765606294911

IPSOS (2021). *Firefighters, healthcare workers and first responders top list of most trusted professions.* https://www.ipsos.com/en-us/news-polls/firefighters-healthcare-workers-and-first-responders-top-list-most-trusted-professions

Janoff-Bulman, R. (1989). Assumptive worlds and the stress of traumatic events: Application of the schema construct. *Social Cognition, 7,* 113–136. doi:10.1521/soco.1989.7.2.113

Joseph, S., Murphy, D., & Regel, S. (2015). Post-traumatic growth in police officers: Guidelines for facilitating post-traumatic growth. In S. M. F. Clevenger, L. Miller, B. A. Moore, & A. Freeman (Eds.), *Behind the badge: A psychological treatment handbook for law enforcement officers* (2015-00709-014; pp. 256–268). Routledge/Taylor & Francis Group. http://ezproxy.tamusa.idm.oclc.org/login?url=https://search.ebscohost.com/login.aspx?direct=true&db=psyh&AN=2015-00709-014&site=ehost-live&scope=site

Karaffa, K. M., & Koch, J. M. (2016). Stigma, pluralistic ignorance, and attitudes toward seeking mental health services among police officers. *Criminal Justice and Behavior, 43*, 759–777. APA PsycInfo. doi:10.1177/0093854815613103

Kunst, M. J. J., Saan, M. C., Bollen, L. J. A., & Kuijpers, K. F. (2017). Secondary traumatic stress and secondary posttraumatic growth in a sample of Dutch police family liaison officers. *Stress and Health: Journal of the International Society for the Investigation of Stress, 33*, 570–577. doi:10.1002/smi.2741

Leppma, M., Mnatsakanova, A., Sarkisian, K., Scott, O., Adjeroh, L., Andrew, M. E., Violanti, J. M., & McCanlies, E. C. (2018). Stressful life events and posttraumatic growth among police officers: A cross-sectional study. *Stress and Health: Journal of the International Society for the Investigation of Stress, 34*, 175–186. doi:10.1002/smi.2772

Linley, P. A., & Joseph, S. (2004). Positive change following trauma and adversity: A review. *Journal of Traumatic Stress, 17*, 11–21. doi:10.1023/B:JOTS.0000014671.27856.7e

McCanlies, E. C., Mnatsakanova, A., Andrew, M. E., Burchfiel, C. M., & Violanti, J. M. (2014). Positive psychological factors are associated with lower PTSD symptoms among police officers: Post Hurricane Katrina. *Stress and Health: Journal of the International Society for the Investigation of Stress, 30*, 405–415. doi:10.1002/smi.2615

McCormack, L., & Riley, L. (2016). Medical discharge from the "family," moral injury, and a diagnosis of PTSD: Is psychological growth possible in the aftermath of policing trauma? *Traumatology, 22*, 19–28. doi:10.1037/trm0000059

McNally, R. J. (2010). Can we salvage the concept of psychological trauma? *The Psychologist, 23*, 386–389. https://psycnet.apa.org/record/2010-10859-002

Mehta, D., Bruenig, D., Pierce, J., Sathyanarayanan, A., Stringfellow, R., Miller, O., Mullens, A. B., & Shakespeare-Finch, J. (2022). Recalibrating the epigenetic clock after exposure to trauma: The role of risk and protective psychosocial factors. *Journal of Psychiatric Research, 149*, 374–381. doi:10.1016/j.jpsychires.2021.11.026

Mennicke, A. M., & Ropes, K. (2016). Estimating the rate of domestic violence perpetrated by law enforcement officers: A review of methods and estimates. *Aggression and Violent Behavior, 31*, 157–164. doi:10.1016/j.avb.2016.09.003

Moore, B. A., Tedeschi, R. G., & Greene, T. C. (2020). A preliminary examination of a posttraumatic growth-based program for veteran mental health. *Practice Innovations*, 1–13. doi:10.1037/pri0000136

Paton, D. (2005). Posttraumatic growth in protective services professionals: Individual, cognitive and organizational influences. *Traumatology, 11*, 335–346. doi:10.1177/153476560501100411

Paton, D. (2006). Critical incident stress risk in police officers: Managing resilience and vulnerability. *Traumatology, 12*, 198–206. doi:10.1177/1534765606296532

Paton, D., & Burke, K. J. (2007). Personal and organizational predictors of posttraumatic adaptation and growth in police officers. *Australasian Journal of Disaster and Trauma Studies, 2007*(1). http://ezproxy.tamusa.idm.oclc.org/login?url=https://search.ebscohost.com/login.aspx?direct=true&db=psyh&AN=2008-10866-005&site=ehost-live&scope=site

Pole, N., Kulkarni, M., Bernstein, A., & Kaufmann, G. (2006). Resilience in retired police officers. *Traumatology, 12*, 207–216. doi:10.1177/1534765606294993

Police Executive Research Forum. (2021). *Survey on Police Workforce Trends.* https://www.policeforum.org/workforcesurveyjune2021

Prokupecz, S., Friedman, M.J., Clarke, R., & Sanchez, R. (November 6, 2022). How the law enforcement response to the Uvalde massacre unfolded as children made chilling 911 calls from inside. *CNN.* https://edition.cnn.com/2022/11/06/us/uvalde-911-classroom-calls/index.html

Schafer, K., Sutter, R., & Gibbons, S. (2015). *Characteristics of individuals and employment among first responders.* U.S. Department of Labor. https://www.hsdl.org/c/view?docid=803088

Shakespeare-Finch, J. E., & Lurie-Beck, J. (2014). A meta-analytic clarification of the relationship between posttraumatic growth and symptoms of posttraumatic distress disorder. *Journal of Anxiety Disorders, 28*, 223–229. APA PsycInfo. doi:10.1016/j.janxdis.2013.10.005

Shochet, I. M., Shakespeare-Finch, J., Craig, C., Roos, C., Wurfl, A., Hoge, R., Young, R. McD., & Brough, P. (2011). The development and implementation of the Promoting Resilient Officers (PRO) Program. *Traumatology, 17*, 43–51. doi:10.1177/1534765611429080

Snell, D. L., Surgenor, L. J., Dorahy, M. J., & Hay-Smith, E. J. C. (2014). Coping and adjustment in New Zealand Police staff 12–18 months after the Canterbury earthquakes: A directed qualitative content analysis. *New Zealand Journal of Psychology, 43*, 5–13.

Tedeschi, R.G., & Calhoun, L.G. (2004). Posttraumatic Growth: Conceptual Foundations and Empirical Evidence. *Psychological Inquiry, 15*, 1–18.

Tedeschi, R. G., Calhoun, L. G., & Groleau, J. M. (2015). Clinical Applications of Posttraumatic Growth. In S. Joseph (Ed.), *Positive Psychology in Practice* (pp. 503–518). John Wiley & Sons, Inc. doi:10.1002/9781118996874.ch30

Tedeschi, R. G., & McNally, R. J. (2011). Can we facilitate posttraumatic growth in combat veterans? *American Psychologist, 66*, 19–24. doi:10.1037/a0021896

U.S. Senate, Committee on Homeland Security and Governmental Affairs. (2019). *Expressing support for the designation of October 28, 2019, as "Honoring the Nation's First Responders Day."* https://www.congress.gov/congressional-report/116th-congress/senate-report/43/1?overview=closed

Violanti, J. M., Hartley, T. A., Gu, J. K., Fekedulegn, D., Andrew, M. E., & Burchfield, C. M. (2013). Life Expectancy in Police Officers: A Comparison with the U.S. General Population. *International Journal of Emergency Mental Health*, *15*, 217–228. https://www.ncbi.nlm.nih.gov/pmc/articles/PMC4734369/

Violanti, J., & Steege, A. (2020). Law enforcement worker suicide: an updated national assessment. *Policing: An International Journal.* doi:10.1108/PIJPSM-09-2019-0157

Wang, Z., Inslicht, S. S., Metzler, T. J., Henn-Haase, C., McCaslin, S. E., Tong, H., Neylan, T. C., & Marmar, C. R. (2010). A prospective study of predictors of depression symptoms in police. *Psychiatry Research*, *175*, 211–216. APA PsycInfo. doi:10.1016/j.psychres.2008.11.010

Westervelt, E. (2021). *Cops Say Low Morale and Department Scrutiny Are Driving Them Away From The Job.* https://www.npr.org/2021/06/24/1009578809/cops-say-low-morale-and-department-scrutiny-are-driving-them-away-from-the-job

Woody, R. H. (2006). Family Interventions with Law Enforcement Officers. *The American Journal of Family Therapy*, *34*, 95–103. doi:10.1080/01926180500376735

Paramedics

5

Jane Shakespeare-Finch and Paul J. Scully

Lyndal

Lyndal is a 43-year-old paramedic who attended counseling and shared her story of attending a young 12-year-old girl who had collapsed in the playground at school. Upon arriving at the scene Lyndal was required to resuscitate and defibrillate the young girl and transport her to hospital. Lyndal remained at the hospital as the young girl was treated and she was still there when the parents arrived; she spoke briefly with them. The young girl was not able to be resuscitated and passed away shortly after the parents' arrival. After having spoken to the parents she left the hospital. "I was very upset by this experience … I could not help her," Lyndal said.

After leaving the hospital and as she returned to her station, she went via her own daughter's school. Lyndal said that she intentionally did so because she wanted to hug her daughter and tell her she loved her. Her daughter was the same age as the young girl she had treated.

The following day Lyndal did a follow-up at the hospital only to find that the young girl had a congenital heart disorder that was not treatable. Lyndal talked about how she struggled over time with the confronting nature of her work, especially treating children; she had attended several seriously injured children and cot deaths and she was grateful that she had received a call from a peer supporter who chatted with her following this case. She said that early in her career she found it difficult to talk with her husband or friends about cases she attended; this put a barrier between her and her husband and friends but with help from colleagues and peer supporters she had been able to learn to cope better and to do the role which she chose and wanted to continue to do. Of this case, she said, "Even though this was not a very nice case, I have come to realize that I am pleased that we did all we could and in some ways, I am pleased I was the one there to care for her. I think I have become better at coping with difficult cases."

DOI: 10.4324/9781003292807-7

Terms used to describe people who work in prehospital emergency medical care vary globally as does the level of training they receive. In some jurisdictions they are referred to as ambulance officers, others as emergency medical technicians or emergency medical responders. In this chapter we refer to people in this occupation as paramedics. The above vignette goes to the core of the multitude of factors influencing individuals who choose to work as paramedics; a role which places them at risk daily of being impacted due to exposure to potentially traumatizing events. While the majority of research examining paramedic mental health has focused on the prevalence of pathology, a growing body of evidence suggests that most paramedics are resilient to the potential trauma they face, and many more experience PTG than psychopathology (e. g., Shakespeare-Finch et al., 2003).

A key factor proposed to underpin health from a salutogenic perspective is a person's sense of coherence; that is, the extent to which an event is comprehensible, manageable, and meaningful. One study that has examined sense of coherence in paramedics was conducted by Ragger and colleagues (2019). These researchers found that a sense of coherence was significantly and positively related to PTG and negatively related to probable PTSD. Further, they found stress and PTG were independent constructs. In this chapter, we embrace the salutogenic view of mental health. We start with motivations for becoming a paramedic, then review the prevalence of psychopathology in paramedics, and look at the research that has examined resilience and PTG. The chapter concludes with factors, both individual and organizational, that have been found to promote mental health in paramedics.

Motivation to be a Paramedic

There is a better understanding of the role of paramedic work nowadays and why individuals choose to work in this occupation which requires a great deal of emotional control in what many would regard as a difficult almost impossible work setting. In an Australian study, Beyond Blue (2018) found that most employees and almost all volunteers across all sectors of emergency work consider their work to be both meaningful and important; this was particularly relevant in the case of Lyndal, who was very committed to her role as paramedic. Linda Ross and colleagues (2016) conducted a survey of 169 paramedicine students seeking to understand their motivation for studying to become a paramedic. Across the board, the most important motivations for students were that they wanted to help people, to save lives, and that they thought it would be an exciting career. Some of the older respondents also added their desire to give back to the community and to have a secure work role.

Prevalence of Psychiatric Disorders

Whilst paramedics can sustain mental health conditions such as PTSD, depression, and anxiety, the likelihood of such diagnosed disorders in some paramedic organizations is quite low. For example, Scully (2011) reports a rate of 0.03% for psychological injury in an Australian paramedical service. In other organizations, the rate of psychopathology is argued to be much higher than that of the general population. For example, a systematic review and meta-analysis of psychiatric disorders in paramedics reported a prevalence rate of distress at 27%, PTSD at 11%, 15% for depression, and 15% of personnel with anxiety (Petrie et al., 2018). Prevalence rates in this review were found to vary greatly across studies and the authors also noted a trend for decreases in the prevalence of disorder over the past three decades. As the nature of the job has not become any easier, this trend is likely to be a result of increased efforts in some organizations at providing proactive as well as reactive staff support services including psychoeducation and a reduction in organizational stigma toward mental health challenges.

There are also elements within this work setting that may contribute to compassion fatigue; these include shift work and extended work hours, as well as recurrent exposure to critical incidents. Stamm (2010) described compassion fatigue as comprised of two factors; secondary traumatic stress (STS) and burnout. She explained that STS has the same symptoms as PTSD but is caused by bearing witness to the trauma of others rather than being the direct victim. Burnout refers to emotional exhaustion, depersonalization, and a reduced sense of personal accomplishment that can occur for some people as a result of their work role. In a sample of Finnish paramedics, Ericsson and colleagues (2021) explored burnout and STS using Stamm's Professional Quality of Life scale (ProQOL; Stamm, 2010). The rates of STS and burnout were not very high and associations between variables were generally weak. Part of their study sought to investigate if participating in defusing or debriefing (i.e., early post-event facilitated group intervention for those workers directly involved in crit- ical incidents) could mitigate levels of STS and burnout. They found no such association between those who did and those who did not participate in defusing. Conversely, Renkiewicz and Hubble (2021), also using the ProQOL, found 48% of their sample (N=686) of U.S. paramedics likely had compassion fatigue. One in two of the participants in this U.S. study had also contemplated suicide. Clearly, the differences are more about organizational context than they are about the nature of the work role. For example, Renkiewicz and Hubble suggested call type (not number) and shift lengths may be contributing factors to the high levels of com- passion fatigue they found.

Not uncommonly, paramedics also describe the impact of an event as being personalized in so far as attending a case of a deceased child where they may have a child of the same age, or dealing with an event that has personal meaning, for example the death of a loved one, the death of a parent, or in some instances suicide (e.g., Jurisova, 2016). These experiences can contribute to the development of compassion fatigue and the possibility of anxiety, depression, and compromised coping. This is seen in the case of Lyndal; she recognized her daughter in the patient she attended to. It is not uncommon for paramedics to find that they have a strong and intimate connection with people for whom they care.

Resilience

Despite the potential for psychiatric injury in paramedics, much trajectory research focusing on trauma exposure, PTSD, depression, and anxiety has found that resilience is a much more common outcome than mental ill-health (e. g. Bonanno, 2005; Bonanno et al., 2012). Gayton and Lovell (2012) investigated resilience levels and the relationship between resilience, wellbeing, and general health in a group of experienced paramedics (n=146) and paramedicine students (n=73). The research found higher levels of resilience in the experienced cohort and significant positive associations between resilience, wellbeing, and general health. Results suggested that paramedics develop resilience on the job rather than resilient individuals being attracted to the job in the first place.

Mausz and colleagues (2022) examined PTSD scores, depression, anxiety, and resilience in 589 Canadian paramedics just prior to the onset of COVID-19. Similar to other research they found approximately 11% of their sample (98% response rate) met the criteria for probable PTSD, 15% for depression, and 15% for anxiety. However, 90% also reported moderate to high levels of resilience. Having a score indicating a mental health disorder was associated with the 10% of people scoring "low" on the resilience scale. The extremely large response rate in this study provides robust data for this particular context. In the U.S., Austin et al. (2018) examined resilience in a small group (n=54) of paramedics and emergency medical technicians and also found high levels of resilience.

In a very new area of research, Miller and colleagues (2020) examined resilience as well as symptoms of PTSD and PTG in a sample of student paramedics. The research was primarily concerned with identifying epigenetic markers for resilience and PTG to unpack potentially different molecular underpinnings to overt behaviors in different trauma outcomes. The candidate genes chosen to examine were those commonly referred to as stress genes, genes that regulate the biological stress cascade, and have been previously found to be implicated in PTSD: *FKBP5* and *NR3C1*. Consistent with survey research cited above, methylation in the *FKBP5* site cg07485685 predicted PTSD symptom severity and also predicted resilience, albeit in opposite directions. In other words, DNA methylation at this site was associated with increased resilience and reduced PTSD symptom severity. The research also found that resilience scores were significantly associated with seven sites; two on *FKBP5* and five on the *NR3C1* gene, further providing evidence for the regulation of the biological stress cascade after the experience of trauma to return to a level of homeostasis. Molecular research has now started to widen investigations into posttraumatic growth (Miller et al., 2020). In general, research from around the world has grown in the examination of PTG. The importance of this becomes clear in the vignette when Lyndal not only demonstrated resilience towards the experienced event but was able to move beyond the potential trauma to find a way to be grateful that she was the person who was able to care for the patient who subsequently died.

Posttraumatic Growth

Shakespeare-Finch et al. (2003) pointed out that for many paramedics the distressing and sometimes traumatic events that they encounter can act as a catalyst for personal and professional growth. In the first published study of PTG in paramedics, growth was found to be much more likely than symptoms of PTSD. In a subsequent study, Shakespeare-Finch and colleagues (2005) identified that although personality factors such as extraversion and openness to experience were significant predictors of PTG, coping strategies mediated those relationships. These findings are important because coping strategies, and indeed resilience, can be responsive to psychoeducation and interventions.

Austin and colleagues (2018) also measured levels of PTG. Consistent with previous research, they found moderate levels of PTG in their sample, especially in areas of personal strength and the appreciation of life domains of the posttraumatic growth inventory (PTGI; Tedeschi & Calhoun, 1996). In the Miller study (2020), PTG was associated with differential methylation of the key genes regulating the biological stress cascade. This was the first published study to confirm that PTG can be identified through relationships with objective biological markers.

Kang and colleagues (2018) investigated PTG in a sample of 227 Chinese paramedics and the relationship PTG had to resilience and social support. Results demonstrated moderate to high mean levels of PTG with a mean level of nearly 70 (*SD*=15.51) on the PTGI (Tedeschi & Calhoun, 1996). Domains of PTG most strongly endorsed were relating to others, new possibilities, and personal strength. There was no difference found in the demographic variables collected including gender, age, marital status, education, or length of service. Ogińska-Bulik and Kobylarczyk (2015) also examined resiliency and PTG in 80 Polish paramedics who had experienced trauma during their work. They also found high mean levels of PTG with 80% of their sample in the moderate to high PTG range, as well as high levels of resiliency. The highest levels of growth found in the Ogińska-Bulik and Kobylarczyk study were in the areas of positive changes in self-perception and appreciation of life.

While individual responsibility for mental health has its place, Lawn et al. (2020) articulated paramedics' wellbeing needs across four key areas: organizational support; informal support; use of humor; and individual mechanisms to cope such as detachment and external supports. In the following section individual strategies are reviewed, followed by organizational ones.

Negotiating the Challenges – Individual Strategies

With the potential for paramedical work to result in psychiatric injury and in resilience and posttraumatic growth, how do paramedics cope with the work they do and stay well? Alexander and Klein (2001) found that a significant number of paramedics develop a strong sense of skill mastery and emotional mastery with continued exposure to cases. They report that this does not suggest that the events are not difficult to deal with or that personnel do not perceive a high level of ongoing distress, but that most paramedics retain a capacity to continue at a high level of professional functioning. In the Oginska-Bulik and Kobylarczyk (2015) study, cited above, active coping and planning were found to be the strongest mediators of resilience and PTG, while venting and denial suppressed such outcomes. Jurisova (2016) also investigated coping strategies in a sample of paramedics from the Slovak Republic. Again, active coping and planning were the strongest positive correlates of total PTG scores. These results are consistent with the theory of PTG; in order to realize PTG a person must actively engage with the traumatic material through effortful rumination among other things (Tedeschi et al., 2018).

Consistent with Lawn and colleagues' (2020) review, Regehr and colleagues (2002) suggested that black humor and a capacity to empathize and to attach meaning to an event are instrumental in the ability of paramedics to cope with the work role. An example of the improved coping strategies is revealed in the above vignette where paramedic Lyndal attempted to save the life of the 12-year-old girl. Lyndal benefited from the support she received from work colleagues and professionals to enhance her coping, enabling her to continue in the role which she chose.

Kang and colleagues (2018) found social support had significant and direct effects on PTG and resilience in Chinese paramedics and an indirect effect on PTG through resilience. Data collected included objective and subjective support as well as support seeking. Each type of support was significantly related to PTG and resilience with objective support, that is, support actually received, providing the strongest relationships. Jurisova (2016) also measured seeking instrumental support and emotional support and found positive relationships between these factors and PTG in paramedics from the Slovak Republic.

Prevention/Risk Minimization – Organizational Strategies

Much work has been done to enhance our understanding of the mental health impact of front-line work on paramedics and the benefits of implementing strategies to enhance coping and mental health; it has also highlighted the mental health benefits of interpersonal support, mental health education, and organizational support. Harrison (2019) suggested it is not only the nature of the operational role that is important in mental health but that organizational issues such as poor leadership and a lack of supervisor support have been demonstrated to have negative impacts on paramedic mental health. Coupled with the large variance in rates of mental health challenges paramedics face around the world, organizational context and culture obviously play a role in protecting and promoting mental health in paramedics. It has been successfully argued in the case of Hegarty versus the Queensland Ambulance Service that organizations, where there is a reasonable risk of foreseeable psychiatric injury, have a duty of care to do what they can to protect and promote mental health in their workforces (Freckelton, 2007).

Scully (2011) described a comprehensive proactive and reactive program to support staff in a paramedic organization. Over a period of 20 years at the time of publication, this organization had been committed to research, reflection, and education in a continuous effort to provide proven and effective programs for staff and their families. Whilst this model was developed and modified over years, there is evidence to support its efficacy in a variety of settings. The following key elements include those identified in the Scully (2011) model and factors outlined in the Beyond Blue (2018) report which speaks to the necessity for organizations to put in place mental health risk minimization strategies. These include:

(1) Pre-employment/induction and ongoing mental health and resilience building education.
(2) Peer Support programs.
(3) Access to professional counseling.
(4) Proactive support following high-level critical incidents.
(5) Proactive support following "low profile" but potentially distressing events.
(6) Workplace connection and social support.
(7) Manager and supervisor mental health and incident response education.

Of particular relevance here is the work by Lawn et al. (2020) who discuss the importance of how organizational management acknowledges and responds to events faced by personnel. Lawn and colleagues claim that "interactions between critical incidents and workplace culture and demands have an overwhelming impact on the psychological, physical and social well-being of ambulance personnel" (p.2). This quote highlights a compelling need for organizational proactive strategies and support for staff members. Lawn goes on to say a further factor in this context is social support, referring to care, love, comfort, esteem, and help received from others; the perception that social support and connectivity, if available as required, may be as protective as actually receiving that support; giving support, however, has also been shown to be significantly beneficial to mental health. Shakespeare-Finch and Obst (2011) observed that social support systems may include family and colleagues as well as religious or spiritual beliefs. This should be seen as a further factor in the "wider culture" of such work environments in ensuring that promoting mental health is a priority and that a variety of levels of support are available. In a study of mental health in paramedics a sense of organizational belongingness was the strongest predictor of professional quality of life, minimizing distress and enhancing resilience (Shakespeare-Finch et. al., 2014). Such workplace support may come from peers formally or informally and from supervisors. The important aspect of this research is that the paramedic feels valued, respected, and cared for within the organization.

Peer support programs have become a leading feature for staff members in a variety of organizations. In emergency services staff, Shakespeare-Finch and Scully (2017) and Kaniasty (2005) point out that good social support in the work setting can be enhanced by well-trained, skilled, and respected peer support officers who are available to assist and support personnel following traumatic incidents in the work context. Whilst this concept is related to connectedness, it is more specific in its focus and is especially applicable in the aftermath of significant traumatic events. In a study that drew on expert opinions from around the world, Creamer and colleagues (2012) provided comprehensive guidelines for effective peer supporters and peer support programs that are consistent with those in the model Scully describes. For example, such people need to be carefully selected and trained not just initially but in an ongoing manner. Professional supervision is a useful addition not only to enhance peer supporters' skills but also to ensure their ongoing mental health.

According to Beyond Blue (2018) and Scully (2011), recruit and induction mental health education focusing on coping and self-care strategies are identified as essential in initiating (employee) connectedness within the workplace, and, in particular, promoting access to peer support and counseling proactively in order to improve coping skills and minimize mental health risk. In the past, debriefing and proactive connection with individuals was more specifically related to high-profile and major critical events; paramedics frequently attend non-high-profile but equally distressing events on a daily basis. In an extensive peer-reviewed study Lawn et.al. (2020) pointed out that whilst there is more work to be done, research suggested that "there was support for robust peer support programs and independent counseling services ... for paramedics" (p. 13). There is also extensive evidence in the literature reviews by Lawn et.al. (2020) and Beyond Blue (2018) supporting the need for the provision of more organizational mental health support and strategies (including Peer Support) to improve workplace connection, access to mental health services, and to reduce work-related stress.

Conclusion

Exposure to critical incidents in combination with complex organizational factors can compromise the mental and physical health and social wellbeing of paramedics. A primary feature of this chapter has been to detail these key issues and to articulate evidence supporting the need for both proactive and reactive support interventions on the part of employers, and to expand carefully constructed workplace-appropriate peer support and mental health education strategies. Importantly, despite strong evidence for a high motivation to enter this particular work role and a general consensus amongst paramedical professionals that they enjoy this work, they are not immune from the impact of distressing incidents. Therefore, organizations have to have in place a comprehensive, proactive, and reactive support program and mental health education strategies. Providing a salutogenic approach, the chapter has not only examined the large variety of prevalence rates for psychiatric disorders in paramedics but also documented the more common outcome of resilience. Perhaps most importantly, the chapter has outlined the potential for this work to also be a catalyst for posttraumatic growth and provided ways in which that growth may be promoted.

References

Alexander, D., & Klein, S. (2001). Ambulance Personnel and critical incidents: The impact of accident and emergency work on mental health. *British Journal of Psychiatry, 17*, 76–81. doi:10.1192/bjp.178.1.76

Austin, C. L., Pathak, M., & Thompson, S. (2018). Secondary traumatic stress and resilience among EMS. *Journal of Paramedic Practice, 10*(6), 240–247 doi:10.12968/jpar.2018.10.6.240

Beyond Blue (2018*).* Answering the Call. National Survey on Police and Emergency Services Final Report. https://research-repository.uwa. edu.au/en/publications/answering-the-call-national-survey-bey ond-blues-national-mental-h?utm_source=nationaltribune&utm_ medium=nationaltribune&utm_campaign=news

Bonanno, G. (2005). Resilience in the face of trauma. *Current Directions in Psychological Science, 14*, 135–138. doi:10.1111/j.0963-7214.2005.00347.x

Bonanno, G. A., Kennedy, P., Galatzer-Levy, I. R., Lude, P., & Elfström, M. L. (2012). Trajectories of resilience, depression, and anxiety following spinal cord injury. *Rehabilitation Psychology*, *57*, 236–247. doi:10.1037/a0029256

Creamer, M., Varker, T., Bisson, J., Darte, K., Greenberg, N., Lau, W., Moreton, G., O'Donnell, M., Richardson, D., Ruzek, J., Watson, P., & Forbes, D. (2012). Guidelines for peer support in high-risk organizations: An international consensus study using the Delphi method. *Journal of Traumatic Stress Studies*, *25*, 134–141. doi:10.1002/jts.21685

Ericsson, C. R., Nordquist, H., Lindström, V. & Rudman, A. (2021). Finnish paramedics' professional quality of life and associations with assignment experiences and defusing use – a cross-sectional study. *BMC Public Health*, *21*, 1789. doi:10.1186/s12889-021-11851-0

Freckelton, I. (2007). Employer's duties for reasonably foreseeable psychiatric injuries. *Psychiatry, Psychology and Law*, *15*, 17–24. doi:10.1080/13218710801979092

Gayton, S. D., & Lovell, G. P. (2012). Resilience in ambulance service paramedics and its relationship with well-being and general health. *Traumatology*, *18*, 58–64. doi:10.1177/1534765610393727

Harrison, J. (2019). Organisational factors: impacting on health for ambulance personnel. *International Journal of Emergency Services*, *8*, 134–146. doi:10.1108/IJES-02-2018-0013

Jurisova, E. (2016). Coping strategies and posttraumatic growth in paramedics: Moderating effect of specific self-efficacy and positive/negative affectivity. *Studia Psychologica*, *58*, 259–275. doi:10.21909sp.2016.04.722

Kang, X., Fang, Y., Li, S., Liu, Y., Zhao, D., Feng, X., Wang, Y., & Li, P. (2018). The benefits of indirect exposure to trauma: the relationships among vicarious posttraumatic growth, social support, and resilience in ambulance personnel in China. *Psychiatry Investigations*, *15*, 452–459. doi:10.30773/pi.2017.11.08.1

Kaniasty, K. (2005). Social support and traumatic stress. *PTSD Research Quarterly,16*, The National Centre for PTSD. https://www.hsdl.org/?view&did=13434

Lawn, S., Roberts, L., Wills, E., Couzner, L., Mohammadi, L., & Goble, E. (2020). The effects of emergency medical service work on the psychological, physical, and social well-being of ambulance personnel: a systematic review of qualitative research. *BMC Psychiatry*, *20*(1), 1–16. doi:10.1186/s12888-020-02752-4

Mausz, J., Donnelly, E. A., Moll, S., Harms, S., & McConnell, M. (2022). Mental disorder symptoms and the relationship with resilience among paramedics in a single Canadian site. *International Journal of Environmental Research and Public Health*, *19*, 4879. doi:10.3390/ijerph19084879

Miller, O., Shakespeare-Finch, J., Bruenig, D., & Mehta, D. (2020). DNA Methylation of *NR3C1* and *FKBP5* predicts Posttraumatic Stress Disorder, Posttraumatic Growth and Resilience. *Psychological Trauma: Research, Theory Practice & Policy*, advance online publication. doi:10.1037/tra0000574

Ogińska-Bulik, N., & Kobylarczyk, M. (2015). Relation between resiliency and post-traumatic growth in a group of paramedics: The mediating role of coping strategies. *International Journal of Occupational Medicine and Environmental Health, 28*, 707–719. doi:10.13075/ijomeh.1896.00323

Petrie, K., Milligan-Saville, J., Gayed, A., Deady, M., Phelps, A., Dell, L., Forbes, D., Bryant, R. A., Calvo, R. A., Glozier, N., & Harvey, S. B. (2018). Prevalence of PTSD and common mental disorders amongst ambulance personnel: a systematic review and meta-analysis. *Social Psychiatry and Psychiatric Epidemiology, 53*, 897–909. doi:10.1007/s00127-018-1539-5

Ragger, K., Hiebler-Ragger, M., Herzog, G., Kapfhammer, H., & Unterrainer, H. (2019). Sense of coherence is linked to post-traumatic growth after critical incidents in Austrian ambulance personnel. *BMC Psychiatry, 19*. doi:10.1186/s12888-019-2065-z

Regehr, C., Goldberg, G., & Hughes, J. (2002). Exposure to human tragedy, empathy, and trauma in ambulance paramedics. *American Journal of Orthopsychiatry, 72*(4), 505–513. doi:10.1037/0002-9432.72.4.505

Renkiewicz, G. K., & Hubble, M. W. (2021). Secondary Traumatic Stress in Emergency Services Systems (STRESS) project: quantifying and predicting compassion fatigue in emergency medical services personnel. *Prehospital Emergency Care, 26*(5). doi:10.1080/10903127.2021.1943578

Ross, L., Hannah, J., & Van Huizen, P. (2016). What motivates students to pursue a career in paramedicine? *Australian Journal of Paramedicine*, 13, 1–8. doi:10.33151/ajp.13.1.484

Scully, P. J. (2011). Taking care of staff: A comprehensive model of support for paramedics and emergency medical dispatchers. *Traumatology, 17*, 35–42. doi:10.1177/1534765611430129

Shakespeare-Finch, J. E., Gow, K, M., & Smith, S. G. (2005). Personality, coping and posttraumatic growth in emergency ambulance personnel. *Traumatology, 11*, 325–334. doi:10.1177/153476560501100410

Shakespeare-Finch, J. E., Smith, S. G., Gow, K. M., Embleton, G., & Baird, I., (2003). The prevalence of posttraumatic growth in emergency ambulance personnel. *Traumatology, 9*, 58–70. doi:10.1177/153476560300900104

Shakespeare-Finch, J., & Obst, P. L. (2011). Development of the 2-Way Social Scale: A measure of giving and receiving, emotional and instrumental support. *Journal of Personality Assessment, 93*, 483–490. doi:10.1080/00223891.2011.594124

Shakespeare-Finch, J., & Scully, P. (2017). Psychosocial Aspects of Disaster Management. In G. Fitzgerald, M. Tarrant, P. Aitken, & M.

Fredriksen (Eds.) *Disaster Health Management: A Primer for Students and Practitioners* (pp. 243–252). Routledge

Shakespeare-Finch, J., Wehr, T., Kaiplinger, I., & Daley, E. (2014). Caring for emergency service personnel: Does what we do work? Proceedings of the Australia & New Zealand Disaster & Emergency Conference, Gold Coast (QLD), 5th–7th May 2014

Stamm, B. H. (2010). *The Concise ProQOL Manual*, 2nd Ed. Pocatello, Copyright © Beth Hudnall Stamm

Tedeschi, R. G., & Calhoun, L. G. (1996). The Posttraumatic Growth Inventory: Measuring the positive legacy of trauma. *Journal of Traumatic Stress, 9*, 455–472. doi:10.1002/jts.2490090305

Tedeschi, R. G., Shakespeare-Finch, J., Taku, K., & Calhoun, L. G. (2018). *Posttraumatic Growth: Theory, Research and Applications.* New York, NY: Routledge

Firefighters

6

Robyn Kirby

Simon

Simon is a 46-year-old Firefighter with over 18 years of service. He phoned the Fire Service counselling line two weeks after attending a training session facilitated by a Counsellor. Simon started the conversation by stating, "My wife has encouraged me to talk to someone, and I saw you at the training a few weeks ago. Is it ok that I talk to you?" Simon explained that he has been experiencing emotions with an intensity that is unfamiliar to him, and that he has recently been 'drinking more than usual.' Simon described shock and embarrassment that he was 'angry and then crying for no reason,' and he voiced concerns that 'I don't understand why I am like this.' In the course of the conversation, Simon spoke about responding to a series of critical incidents over the past month and realized that some details of these events had 'stuck' with him. One was a motor vehicle accident involving a pregnant woman who died at the scene, and another incident was a young man who had committed suicide by hanging. Simon referred to initial feelings of anger regarding the suicide – upon deeper reflection facilitated by the Counsellor, Simon identified feeling devastated that someone chose to take their own life, and referred to the incidents being 'such a waste.' Simon shared personal family history – he is married and has a very supportive wife who is concerned about his increased drinking and social 'withdrawal.' They have a 23-year-old daughter with whom they enjoy a very close relationship. The confidential conversation with the Counsellor allowed Simon to safely express his emotions and explore the application of some adaptive coping strategies. Coincidentally, at the start of his next shift Simon was approached by his Station Leader, who enquired about his wellbeing after noticing that Simon was 'out of character lately.' The Chief's actions are an example of supportive leadership assuming an active role to intervene with early signs of behavior change. Following their chat, the Station Leader arranged ongoing support through the local Peer Support Officer (PSO), and Simon (and his family) sincerely appreciated the range of support

DOI: 10.4324/9781003292807-8

provided. He commented that the experience has inspired him to consider becoming a PSO in the future.

The Firefighter role demands physical, mental, and emotional strength. Firefighters are highly respected for their role in front-line response to emergency and disaster events, to defend people, property, and environment from harm. In this chapter, the description of 'Firefighter' encompasses all who assume this role. It incorporates those who volunteer to help during times of large-scale bush or wildfire events, those who may be employed on a "part-time" or "casual" basis, and those who consider themselves to be "career" Firefighters, paid fulltime to perform the role. In some countries, a Firefighter's role is engaged with a broad range of emergency situations, and in other cases the role is explicitly to respond to a fire event (Cook & Mitchell, 2013). Each role and situation may present some unique challenges, however there are also some universal risks and needs to be considered in relation to mental health and wellbeing. The above vignette captures some of the themes that may influence the mental health outcomes for Firefighters.

Context of frontline Fire and Emergency Services

Firefighters work under difficult circumstances with long work hours and frequent exposure to high stress situations and potentially traumatic events. Different specialisations within the fire department may be at an even more increased risk of psychological harm due to extended exposures to potentially challenging scenes. Firefighters' work schedules are typically based on a shift work roster comprising four shifts of two x 10-hour days and two x 14-hour night shifts, followed by four days off. In some countries, the shift may extend for 24-hour periods, where Firefighters work, eat, and sleep (when possible) at the Fire Station (Billings & Focht, 2016). Part-time or 'Auxiliary' Firefighters are generally employed in external roles and respond to emergency Fire Service calls on an "as needed" basis with potentially short notice. Fire Services are often reliant upon a strong foundation of volunteers, especially in rural and remote areas, who donate their time and skills to protect lives and property from fires, as well as provide preventative education for community safety (Beyond Blue, 2018a).

In addition to responding to fires, Firefighters may also conduct rescues from motor vehicle accidents, provide rescue and recovery during disaster events, perform first aid and medical assistance, contain toxic hazards, and assist with suicide intervention. Other specialist roles such as "Technical Rescue" involve elevated danger due to rescues from precarious positions such as heights, swift moving water, confined spaces, or hazardous materials. Urban Search and Rescue technicians are often deployed to rescue people involved with mass casualty events including earthquakes and tsunamis. The role of Fire Investigator poses some additional challenges due to the intense and prolonged exposure to a high-risk environment. Fire Investigators need to determine the contributing factors of a fatal house fire, which could involve spending extended time sifting through the remains of someone's home, closely examining artefacts, surrounded by their personal belongings and potentially grieving relatives or community members, whilst also managing forensic reports and media attention to high-profile events. Each of these circumstances increase the level of exposure to potentially traumatic experiences, and therefore need to be considered when formulating the organizational support response.

Mental health of Firefighters

Responding to crisis, disasters, and large-scale mass trauma events is a challenging work environment inherent in Firefighter duties. These events can escalate stress reactions and may accumulate over time which increases risk of developing mental health conditions (Beyond Blue, 2018a; Cook & Mitchell, 2013). Posttraumatic stress disorder (PTSD) continues to be the most widely researched topic in first responder literature. Studies report significant variance in the prevalence rates of PTSD among Firefighters, with global figures ranging from 6.5% to 37% (Cook & Mitchell, 2013; Laureys & Easton, 2020). An Australian study of mental health of first responders in 2018 cites a prevalence rate of around 9% of Firefighters experiencing PTSD symptoms (Beyond Blue, 2018a). Indirect exposure to trauma, or cumulative experience with multiple traumatic events, may be associated with mental health conditions such as vicarious trauma, secondary trauma, compassion fatigue, and burn out (Haslam & Mallon, 2003).

However, it is important to recognize that PTSD is not the only mental health outcome that may arise following a traumatic experience. As mentioned in other chapters in this book, emergency services personnel generally report higher rates of resilience and posttraumatic growth outcomes than psychological injury following exposure to trauma. Whilst events may be distressing, many Firefighters acknowledge that the role also creates opportunity for personal and professional growth. Substantial research has identified that most people recover well with some basic support from friends and family (Bonnano et al., 2010; Phoenix, 2020). Furthermore, they may also experience positive outcomes as a result of the difficult experience, which is often described as posttraumatic growth (Tedeschi et al., 2018).

Fortunately, research is increasingly recognizing the need to examine the factors that contribute to positive outcomes, such as resilience and posttraumatic growth, which assists organizations to employ initiatives that promote wellbeing from a strengths-based perspective. Adopting this approach acknowledges the diversity of individual strengths, cultural influences, and organizational protective factors that will positively influence mental health and wellbeing (Cook & Mitchell, 2013; Counson et al., 2019; Shakespeare-Finch, 2007).

Psychosocial Risks and Protective factors

Unpredictable and challenging environments

Emergency situations often present unpredictable situations in which Firefighters find themselves performing tasks not common to their role. This poses a risk to wellbeing, in that Firefighters moral values may provoke responsibility to assist, even when they do not have the resources and/or specific training for the task (Phoenix, 2020). Whilst this highlights their ingenuity and resourcefulness, if the outcome does not successfully save life, it can escalate stress and leave Firefighters with feelings of being ill-prepared which impact on mental health. In 2007, Perrin and colleagues undertook a study investigating differences in PTSD prevalence among various occupations involved with the rescue and recovery of the World Trade Centre disaster. The researchers identified that PTSD was significantly higher among those who performed tasks outside of their usual scope. Additionally, the cumulative exposure of multiple trauma experiences can take a toll on mental health over time (Beyond Blue, 2018a; Cook & Mitchell, 2013).

Gender differences

Even though the gender balance has changed over time, at present, Fire Services typically report a higher ratio of males in the occupation. Figures range from 2% to 20% of female Firefighters, with the New Zealand Fire Service claiming the highest proportion of women involved with Volunteer Firefighting (Fire & Emergency New Zealand, 2020). Research exploring gender differences in relation to mental health has found that males in general, and Firefighters specifically, are inclined to use alcohol and humor as a way of distracting or avoiding thoughts and feelings associated with difficult experiences (Cook & Mitchell, 2013; Haddock et al., 2012; Poston et al., 2013). This maladaptive coping strategy of escapism, avoidance, and using substances to numb emotions was seen in Simon's case, and was one of the behavior changes that instigated him to access additional support.

Shift work

As outlined earlier, work schedules for Firefighters are based on shiftwork patterns which are disruptive to the body's natural circadian rhythm. Furthermore, Firefighters often sleep in the station under conditions that are not conducive to good quality sleep, such as flashing lights and turn out alarms (Cook & Mitchell, 2013). Studies investigating sleep quality among Firefighters have identified over 70% report poor sleep, and this is reportedly worse for those who maintain secondary employment on their "days off" (Billings & Focht, 2016; Haslom & Mallon, 2003; Isaac & Buchannan, 2021). A systematic review by Frost and colleagues (2021) found that poor sleep negatively impacted cognitive performance, but not the physical capabilities of Firefighters. A study examining interactions between Firefighters' work roles, sleep, and personal relationships, found that Firefighters and their family members described challenges of poor communication and being emotionally unavailable in the immediate period following their work shift (Watkins et al., 2021). With sleep known to be strongly linked to mental wellbeing, this presents an important rationale for managing sleep and fatigue.

Physical and Mental Fitness

Firefighters generally maintain a high level of fitness to perform their role. Physical activity is recommended as a technique to assist with reducing arousal (adrenalin) following a high stress event. Whilst this may occur naturally during the performance of routine work-related tasks (e.g., cleaning and repacking of equipment), it can also be intentionally achieved through gym workout when time permits (Haslam & Mallon, 2003; Phoenix, 2020).

Additionally, their selection, training, and induction provides opportunity to hone skills for mental fitness. Firefighters often report using a cognitive strategy to maintain a task-oriented focus and situational awareness during operational response. Research suggests that this focuses the mind towards actions required to facilitate the best chance of success for the rescue operation, which naturally diminishes emotional reactions at the time. It is important for Firefighters to have an awareness of their reactions, as well as skills and resources to manage these reactions in the short and long term (Laureys & Easton, 2020; Phoenix, 2020; van Hoof et al., 2017).

Organizational Strategies and Support Services

Whilst there is an increased risk of exposure to trauma, there are also a number of protective factors and organizational strategies that positively influence wellbeing. Workplace health and safety legislation in many countries outlines organizations' responsibilities for the safety of their workforce, including psychological safety. Most organizations adopt a rigorous recruitment and selection process, as well as training and induction processes to successfully perform their role, including preparation for managing the psychosocial aspects of potentially traumatic events (Beyond Blue, 2018b; WHO, 2022).

Simon's situation demonstrates that, even with robust training processes and experience, there are times when aspects of the situation can become emotionally overwhelming. This can occur for many reasons, some of them related to the individual and pre-existing vulnerabilities, others due to the circumstances of the event, and often influenced by the support that is (or is not) received after. In Simon's case, the conversation with the counsellor uncovered elements of the event that he had personalized – the young man who committed suicide was of similar age to his daughter. It is common for people to experience escalated arousal when they feel a direct connection with the traumatic event. However, Simon had not shared any of these concerns with anyone, which contributed to his feeling overwhelmed and caused him to isolate and withdraw from others with feelings of shame. This describes a common barrier to Firefighters seeking help – referred to as "stigma."

Stigma

There are many reasons why people are discouraged from talking about their experience and seeking help. This can include "stigma" or fear of how they may be judged by others, worry that they may be perceived negatively which may limit career progression, or circumstances may prevent people from having a suitable opportunity to do so. Additionally, people may impose "self-stigma" through thoughts of "not wanting to let the team down," and feelings of shame can prevent them from reaching out for assistance (Beyond Blue, 2018a; Isaac & Buchannan, 2021; Phoenix, 2020).

A meta-analysis by Haugen et al. (2017) outlined several barriers to first responders seeking help, for example, concerns about confidentiality, scheduling concerns, and lack of knowing where to get help. Delaying assistance poses a risk of increased symptoms, which highlights the need for organizational strategies that encourage people to seek help sooner to promote faster recovery (Beyond Blue, 2018b; van Hoof et al., 2017; WHO, 2022). Confidentiality and accessibility of support services are crucial, as well as the importance of routinely educating people about the support options available to them (Beyond Blue 2018b; WHO, 2022). Some of these barriers were evident in Simon's case. Fortunately, Simon was able to overcome his initial concerns with some encouragement from his wife and recent positive interaction with the counsellor, which prompted him to reach out for support.

Family support

It is important to think broadly about the possible effects of trauma. Research into the impacts of their service on Firefighters' families is limited, although it is a common concern among Firefighters. Family members may experience fear and worry about their loved one who may be working in dangerous conditions, as well as pressures and frustrations with the shift work lifestyle. Hence, support services need to be made available and family members made aware of the support options accessible to them (Cook & Mitchell, 2013). The New Zealand Fire Service addressed this issue with a creative and novel initiative, by sourcing an author to design a children's book which serves as a resource to generate conversations among family members about the challenges of the firefighter role (New Zealand Firefighters Charity, 2022).

Family members are often the initial and preferred source of support for Firefighters, and therefore would benefit from having a basic knowledge of support resources and referral options (Laureys & Easton, 2020). This information provides useful context for organizations to consider utilizing family members as sources of indirect support that have a strong influence on Firefighters' wellbeing. Organizations can provide education, resources, and support to Firefighter's families to assist them in managing the unique challenges and impact on family life, as well as an early form of intervention to encourage their loved one to access additional support as needed (Cherry et al., 2021; Phoenix, 2020). However, some Firefighters may not have opportunity for this source of support, and/or are inclined to "protect" family from their work stressors. In such cases, support from peers and colleagues becomes increasingly important (Cook & Mitchell, 2013; Laureys & Easton, 2020).

Psychosocial support

Research cites absence of social support as the largest risk for developing PTSD symptoms (Van Hoof et al., 2017). According to models of resilience and posttraumatic growth, psychosocial support is a variable that positively influences some of the cognitive processes such as deliberate rumination (Tedeschi & Calhoun, 2016), and is a significant factor in achieving mental wellbeing (Haslam & Mallon, 2003). Studies identifying Firefighters' preferences for support has suggested that support from family and friends is highly favored, however there are also occasions when this was not considered appropriate. Informal support from colleagues is also highly rated, with humor and shared experience among colleagues creating an increased sense of social connection, belongingness, and job satisfaction (Haslam & Mallon, 2003; Laureys & Easton, 2020). Longitudinal studies with Canadian Firefighters found that social support from peers assisted with reducing symptoms of occupational stress, and also addressed some of the barriers associated with stigma (Isaac & Buchanan, 2022). Another study compared mental health outcomes following a traumatic event and noted that peer support was associated with a marked reduction in cases of anxiety, depression, and PTSD symptoms, even after several months following the event (Cherry et al., 2021).

Further research among U.S. Firefighters sought to explore variations between the source of support from supervisors, co-workers, or family/friends, and found support initiated by their supervisor was especially valuable (Stanley et al., 2019). This emphasizes the powerful role that Leaders play in managing mental health and wellbeing. A common theme within all of these studies is that Firefighters appreciated all forms of support, and ideally favored having a range of options to draw upon. This is consistent with resilience and psychosocial models that recommend empowering people with personal choice in their recovery (Beshai & Carleton, 2016; Cook & Mitchell, 2013).

Following the Australian "Black Summer" Bushfires, a research study examined volunteer Firefighters' experience with wellbeing support and advocated for proactive, reactive, and an holistic approach (Smith et al., 2022). Organizations can foster opportunities for social support, valuable connection, and constructive discussion which can help gain an objective perspective and process the experience. There is limited support for the effectiveness of single session critical incident stress debriefing (CISD) in reducing posttraumatic psychopathology (McNally et al., 2003; Rose et al., 2002). Participants in these sessions often subjectively report the intervention as helpful, although there appears to be no effect on PTSD symptoms (Bisson et al., 2007; McNally et al., 2003).

However, there is also argument for benefits of group support that provides safe opportunity for emotional expression, cognitive processing, and psychosocial support that assists individual and community recovery (McNally, 2003; Rose et al., 2002; Phoenix, 2020). Studies with first responders have acknowledged a strong sense of group cohesion and preference for support in a group format (Phoenix, 2020). Whilst research continues to evaluate and debate the value of psychosocial interventions following traumatic events, the current recommendation is that post-trauma support should adopt a range of evidence-informed approaches that aim to respect individual needs and preferences for recovery (McNally, 2003; Phoenix, 2020).

Resilience and Posttraumatic Growth (PTG)

In the early days of trauma research, the focus centered on PTSD as the primary outcome. Since then, a host of research has sought to explore the factors that contribute to healthy adjustment, resilience, and personal growth after adversity (Bonnano et al., 2010; Kirby et al., 2011; Shakespeare-Finch, 2007; Tedeschi et al., 2018). Research to date suggests that a person is more likely to experience PTG following a traumatic event when they engage in adaptive, problem-solving coping and deliberate rumination with the intention to understand and process a traumatic experience (Kirby et al., 2011; Tedeschi & Calhoun, 2016). A study of 226 Korean firefighters identified that PTG can be enhanced through deliberate rumination and utilizing problem-focused coping strategies (Yang & Ha, 2019). Australian studies have found a strong sense of comradery among volunteer Firefighters (Tuckey & Hayward, 2011) and social support among paid Firefighters (Armstrong et al., 2016) served as protective factors against posttraumatic symptoms and burnout.

The study by Armstrong and colleagues (2016) cites the factors most strongly linked to PTSD among Firefighters relate to organizational stressors, and PTG was influenced by utilizing "self-care" coping strategies and having a sense of organizational belongingness. These findings suggest that efforts toward relieving organizational stressors, strengthening organizational belongingness, and fostering adaptive coping among Firefighters may reduce intensity of PTSD symptoms and promote PTG (Armstrong et al, 2016). As outlined by Shakespeare-Finch (2007), some emergency services have shifted away from the pathological approach of providing mental health interventions after psychological problems became apparent to a more proactive, holistic, and salutogenic approach adopting programs aimed at building resilience in individuals and strengthening the psychological support frameworks within organizations.

There are several examples of resilience and PTG in the vignette, which was largely influenced through positive experiences of psychosocial support. Simon was somewhat surprised initially, then grateful for the concern and support of his Station Leader, peers, and family. He was encouraged by his close social network and overcame initial feelings of shame to reach out for help and experienced it to be beneficial. In the process, he learned about his own stress reactions and practical strategies that assist in coping with high stress events. His initial stigma and fears about talking to others were quickly erased by caring colleagues and trusted professionals. This has encouraged Simon to advocate to others the benefits of accessing help, and he has been inspired to learn more about supporting others to become a PSO.

Organizational Strategies

Many countries assume "duty of care," legislative obligations and organizational values that recognize the importance of caring for the safety of staff and volunteers, as well as a social and/or moral responsibility for their wellbeing. Ideally, mental health and wellbeing is a shared responsibility of individuals and organizations (Beyond Blue, 2018b; WHO, 2022). A thematic analysis exploring organizational factors that serve as facilitators or barriers to Firefighters' resilience identified four key themes (Conway & Waring, 2020). Firstly, "informal support" among colleagues influences close working relationships and builds a supportive workplace culture. "Formal support" activities provided by the organization to support firefighters with their mental health and wellbeing were generally perceived positively. "Basic welfare measures" were considered to be a foundation of good leadership and organizational support, and "trust" was believed to be an important influencing factor for Firefighters' willingness to access these resources (Conway & Waring, 2020).

Education, Training and Health promotion opportunities

Psychological preparedness is one of the variables found to improve well-being and increase resilience, which provides a strong rationale for the importance of training and education (Paton, 2006; Shakespeare-Finch, 2007). Training needs to be targeted for specific audiences, address specific needs, encourage early access to seek assistance and be continually offered throughout the Firefighter career span (e.g., recruits, experienced firefighters, promotion stages to Leaders/Managers, tailored for specialist roles or high-risk groups, in preparation for retirement), and at relevant times such as following major incidents or organizational change.

Following the popularity of online digital mental health and psychosocial support applications, a number of emergency service organizations have developed online and "virtual reality" training, as well as phone apps that offer education, emotional regulation, and mindfulness strategies with positive effect. For example, an Australian study by Counson and colleagues (2019) explored the effectiveness of online mindfulness programs and have suggested some benefits in reducing symptoms of depression and anxiety among Firefighters recently exposed to trauma.

With reference to Simon's case, the mental health training provided him with knowledge of the referral options, as well as facilitating familiarity with the Counsellor which helped reduce barriers for Simon to initiate contact when he needed assistance. The positive influence of leader education and support is also evident in Simon's case study. These combined experiences assisted with reducing the stigma of mental health concerns, and facilitated a positive outcome for Simon who is now actively advocating the benefits of accessing support to others.

Support Services

The evidence informed recommendations for high-risk organizations in managing mental health attest that organizations should provide a broad range of support services to meet diverse needs, with a stepped care approach that extends support and treatment as needs escalate (Beyond Blue, 2018b; McFarlane & Bryant, 2007). Many Fire Services use complimentary support services including networks of Chaplains, Peer Support Officers (PSOs), professional Counsellors, specialist Advisors to assist with injury management or conflict situations and change management, and Leader/Manager coaching and support, as well as proactive and reactive support for high risk events such as critical incidents, cumulative incidents/multiple events, and disaster operations through an integrated critical incident management process for early intervention of post-trauma support (Beyond Blue, 2018b; Creamer et al., 2012; Phoenix, 2020).

Another successful organizational initiative to break down barriers of stigma and encourage help-seeking behavior is the sharing of "lived experiences," where Firefighters who have had difficult or challenging life experiences share their personal stories (Beyond Blue, 2018b; Cook & Mitchell, 2013). Peer Support programs are recognized as an important early intervention for mental health in high risk organizations and are evolving as a common intervention strategy among emergency organizations (Beyond Blue, 2018b; Creamer et al., 2012; Phoenix, 2020).

Conclusion

In summary, professional and volunteer Firefighters are routinely exposed to distressing and traumatic incidents, as well as having demanding pressures in their work roles. This poses an increased risk of developing psychological injury (Beyond Blue, 2018a). However, research reports a higher proportion of emergency service personnel experience resilience and PTG, and continues to explore the factors that contribute to these outcomes (Laureys & Easton, 2020; Shakespeare-Finch et al., 2003). This chapter has outlined a number of pertinent issues for consideration when developing an effective organizational intervention to optimize mental health and wellbeing. These initiatives aim to foster a positive workplace culture that values and supports mental health and wellbeing, which will combat stigma and encourage people to access help when needed.

References

Armstrong, D., Shakespeare-Finch, J., & Shochet, I. (2014) Predicting post-traumatic growth and post-traumatic stress in firefighters. *Australian Journal of Psychology, 66*(1), 38–46. doi:10.1111/ajpy.12032

Armstrong, D., Shakespeare-Finch, J., & Shochet, I. (2016). Organizational belongingness mediates the relationship between sources of stress and post-trauma outcomes in firefighters. *Psychological trauma: theory, research, practice, and policy, 8*, 343. doi:10.1037/tra0000083

Beshai, S., & Carleton R. N. (2016). *Peer support and crisis-focused psychological intervention programs in Canadian first responders: Blue Paper.* Regina, SK: University of Regina Collaborative Centre for Justice and Safety. Retrieved 14 November 2022 from http://www.justiceandsafety.ca/resources/cipsrt

Beyond Blue (2018a). Answering the Call. National Survey on Police and Emergency Services Detailed Report. https://www.beyondblue.org.au/docs/default-source/resources/bl1898-pes-full-report_final.pdf

Beyond Blue (2018b). Developing a workplace mental health strategy. A how-to guide for organisations. Sourced from https://www.headsup.org.au/docs/default-source/resources/393615_1117_bl1833_acc-2.pdf

Billings, J., & Focht, W. (2016). Firefighter Shift Schedules Affect Sleep Quality. *Journal of Occupational and Environmental Medicine, 58,* 294–298https://www.jstor.org/stable/48501179

Bisson, J. I., Brayne, M., Ochberg, F. M., & Everly Jr, G. (2007). Early psychosocial intervention following traumatic events. *American Journal of Psychiatry, 164,* 1016–1019. doi:10.1176/ajp.2007.164.7.1016

Bonanno, G. A., Brewin, C. R., Kaniasty, K., & Greca, A. M. L. (2010). Weighing the Costs of Disaster: Consequences, Risks, and Resilience in Individuals, Families, and Communities. *Psychological Science in the Public Interest, 11,* 1–49. doi:10.1177/1529100610387086

Calhoun, L. G., & Tedeschi, R. G. (2006). The foundation of post-traumatic growth: An expanded framework. In L. G. Calhoun & R. G. Tedeschi (Eds.) *Handbook of Posttraumatic Growth: Research and Practice* (pp. 18–64). Lawrence Erlbaum Associates: MahWah, NJ

Cherry, N., Galarneau, J-M., Haynes, W., & Sluggett, B. (2021). The role of organizational supports in mitigating mental ill health in firefighters: a cohort study in Alberta, Canada. *American Journal of Industrial Medicine, 64,* 593–601. doi:10.1002/ajim.23249

Conway, R. R., & Waring, S. (2020). Facilitators and barriers to developing firefighter resilience. *Disaster Prevention and Management, 30,* 327–339. doi:10.1108/DPM-06-2018-0186

Cook, B., & Mitchell, W. (2013). *Occupational health effects for firefighters: The extent and implications of physical and psychological injuries.* Report prepared for the United Firefighters Union of Australia, Victoria Branch. Centre of Full Employment and Equity. https://s3.ap-southeast-2.amazonaws.com/hdp.au.prod.app.vic-engage.files/3914/8609/8798/Attachment_-_UFU_Submission_to_FSR_-_ANNEXURE_59.PDF

Counson, I., Hosemans, D., Lal, T., Mott, B., Harvey, S., & Joyce, S. (2019). Mental health and mindfulness amongst Australian fire fighters. *BMC Psychology, 7*(1). doi:10.1186/s40359-019-0311-2

Creamer, M., Varker, T., Bisson, J., Darte, K., Greenberg, N., Lau, W., Moreton, G., O'Donnell, M., Richardson, D., Ruzek, J., Watson, P., & Forbes, D. (2012). Guidelines for peer support in high-risk organizations: An international consensus study using the Delphi method. *Journal of Traumatic Stress Studies, 25,* 134–141. doi:10.1002/jts.21685

Dean, P. G., Gow, K., & Shakespeare-Finch, J. (2003). Counting the Cost: Psychological Distress in Career and Auxiliary Firefighters. *The Australasian Journal of Disaster and Trauma Studies, 2003-1.* Retrieved from: https://psycnet.apa.org/record/2004-20447-002

Everly Jr., G. S., Lating, J. M., Sherman, M. F., & Goncher, I. (2016). The potential efficacy of psychological first aid on self-reported anxiety and mood: A pilot study. *Journal of Nervous & Mental Disease, 204,* 233–235. doi:10.1097/NMD.0000000000000429

Fire and Emergency New Zealand (2020). *Annual report for the year ending 30 June 2020.* Retrieved 14 November 2022 from: https://www.firea ndemergency.nz/assets/Documents/About-FENZ/Key-documents/ FENZ-Annual-Report-2019-2020.pdf

Frost, C., Toczko, M., Merrigan, J. J., and Martin, J. R. (2021). The effects of sleep on firefighter occupational performance and health: A systematic review and call for action. *Sleep Epidemiology, 1.* doi:10.1016/ j.sleepe.2021.100014

Haddock, C. K., Jahnke, S. A., Poston, W. S., Jitnarin, N., Kaipust, C. M., Tuley, B., & Hyder, M. L. (2012). Alcohol use among firefighters in the Central United States. *Occupational Medicine, 62,* 661–664. doi:10.1093/ occmed/kqs162

Haslam, C., & Mallon, K. (2003). A preliminary investigation of port-traumatic stress symptoms in firefighters. *Work & Stress, 17,* 277–285. doi:10.1080/02678370310001625649

Haugen, P. T., McCrillis, A. M., Smid, G. E., & Nijdam, M. J. (2017). Mental health stigma and barriers to mental health care for first responders: A systematic review and meta-analysis. *Journal of Psychiatric Research, 94,* 218–229. doi:10.1016/j.jpsychires.2017.08.001

Isaac, G. M., & Buchanan, M. J. (2021). Extinguishing Stigma among Firefighters: An Examination of Stress, Social Support, and Help-Seeking Attitudes. *Psychology, 12,* 349–373. doi:10.4236/ psych.2021.123023

Kirby, R., Shakespeare-Finch, J., & Palk, G. (2011). Adaptive and mal-adaptive coping strategies predict post-trauma outcomes in ambu-lance personnel. *Traumatology, 17,* 5–34. doi:10.1177/153476561039562

Laureys, V., & Easton, M. (2020). Resilience of firefighters exposed to potentially traumatic events: a literature review. *International Journal of Emergency Services, 9,* 217–232. doi:10.1108/IJES-05-2019-0021

McFarlane, A. C. & Bryant, R. A. (2007). Post-traumatic stress disorder in occupational settings: anticipating and managing the risk. *Occupational Medicine, 57,* 404–410. doi:10.1093/occmed/kqm070

McNally, R. J., Bryant, R. A., & Ehlers, A. (2003). Does Early Psychological Intervention Promote Recovery From Posttraumatic Stress? *Psychological Science in the Public Interest, 4,* 45–79. doi:10.1111/ 1529-1006.01421

New Zealand Firefighters Charity (2022) *Charity launches free children's book for firefighters' families.* Retrieved from https://www.fire-magazine. com/charity-launches-free-childrens-book-for-firefighters-families

Paton, D. (2006). Posttraumatic growth in emergency professionals. In. L. Calhoun and R. Tedeschi (Eds) *Handbook of Posttraumatic Growth. Research and Practice.* (pp. 225 – 247). Mahwah, MJ: Lawrence Erlbaum Association

Perrin, M., Digrande, L., Wheeler, K., Thorpe, L., Farfel, M., & Brackbill, R. (2007). Differences in PTSD Prevalence and Associated Risk Factors Among World Trade Center Disaster Rescue and Recovery Workers.

The American Journal of Psychiatry, 164, 1385–1394. doi:10.1176/appi. ajp.2007.06101645

Phoenix Australia – Centre for Posttraumatic Mental Health. (2020). *Specific Populations and Trauma Types: Emergency services personnel in Australian Guidelines for the Prevention and Treatment of Acute Stress Disorder, Posttraumatic Stress Disorder and Complex Posttraumatic Stress Disorder.* Phoenix Australia. Retrieved 13 December 2022 from: https://www. phoenixaustralia.org/wp-content/uploads/2022/08/Chapter-9-3.- Emergency-services-personnel-1.pdf

Poston, W. S., Haddock, C. K., Jahnke, S. A., Jitnarin, N., & Day, R. S. (2013). An examination of the benefits of health promotion programs for the national fire service. *BMC Public Health, 13,* 805. doi:10.1186/ 1471-2458-13-805

Rose, S. C., Bisson, J., Churchill, R., & Wessely, S. (2002). Psychological debriefing for preventing post-traumatic stress disorder (PTSD). *Cochrane Database of Systematic Reviews, 2, CD000560.* Retrieved from https://doi.org/10.1002/14651858.CD000560

Shakespeare-Finch, J. (2007). *Building Resilience in Emergency Service Personnel through Organisational Structures.* Proceedings of the 42nd Conference of the Australian Psychological Society. Australian Psychological Society, Australia, pp. 362–365

Smith, E., Holmes, L., Larkin, B., Mills, B., & Dobson, M. (2022). Supporting Volunteer Firefighter Well-Being: Lessons from the Australian "Black Summer" Bushfires. *Prehospital and Disaster Medicine, 37,* 273–276. doi:10.1017/S1049023X22000322

Stanley, I. H., Hom, M. A., Chu, C., Dougherty, S. P., Gallyer, A. J., Spencer-Thomas, S., Shelef, L., Fruchter, E., Comtois, K. A., Gutierrez, P. M., Sachs-Ericsson, N. J., & Joiner, T. E. (2019). Perceptions of belongingness and social support attenuate PTSD symptom severity among firefighters: A multistudy investigation. *Psychological Services, 16,* 543–555. doi:10.1037/ser0000240

Tedeschi, R. G. & Calhoun, L. G. (2016). Posttraumatic Growth. *Encyclopedia of Mental Health, 3,* 305–307. doi:10.1016/B978-0-12-397045-9.00246-9

Tedeschi, R. G., Shakespeare-Finch, J., Taku, K., & Calhoun, L. G. (2018). *Posttraumatic Growth: Theory, Research and Applications.* New York, NY: Routledge

Tuckey, M. R., & Hayward, R. (2011). Global and occupation- specific emotional resources as buffers against the emotional demands of fire-fighting. *Applied Psychology, 60,* 1–23 doi:10.1111/ j.1464-0597.2010.00424.x

van Hoof, M., McFarlane, A., Lawrence-Wood, E., Abraham, M., Bryant, R., & Sim, M. (2017). *South Australian Metropolitan Fire Service (MFS) Health and Wellbeing Study: Executive Report.* https://www.mfs.sa.gov.au/ Warnings,-Media-and-Publications/publications,-plans-and-repo rts/community-information-reporting/mfs-health-and-wellbeing- study/MFS-Health-and-Wellbeing-Study-Executive-Summary.pdf

Watkins, S. L., Shannon, M. A., Hurtado, D. A., Shea, S. A., & Bowles, N. P. (2021). Interactions between home, work, and sleep among firefighters. *American Journal of Industrial Medicine*, *64*, 137–148. doi:10.1002/ajim.23194

World Health Organisation (WHO) (2022). *Guidelines on Mental Health at Work*. Geneva: World Health Organization. Licence: CC BY-NC-SA 3.0 IGO. Cataloguing-in-Publication (CIP) data. Retrieved 8 December 2022 from: https://www.who.int/publications/i/item/9789240053052

Yang, S. K., & Ha, Y. (2019). Predicting Posttraumatic Growth among Firefighters: The Role of Deliberate Rumination and Problem-Focused Coping. *International Journal of Environmental Research and Public Health*, *16*, 3879. doi:10.3390/ijerph16203879

Disaster and Emergency Response Volunteers

7

Leanne Hinsch and James Douglas

Graham

About ten years ago, Graham, a volunteer trained in disaster response, was called to respond to an unprecedented flooding event in his neighbouring community. He had been keen to put into action the water rescue training he did with another organization the year before, but his training hadn't yet been recognised at work, which he found frustrating. He would be tasked with a different role this time. Graham had been eager to receive the authorisation for deployment, feeling helpless while his group waited for the flood waters to recede enough for their search role in the response efforts to be safe. While waiting, he'd heard news about the disaster and wondered if the people he knew from that community were safe or not. An unexpected wall of water that mimicked an inland tsunami left the entire town inundated to the roofs of houses within minutes. There had hardly been any warning. As a park ranger in his full-time position, he knew this area well and couldn't imagine the gravity of the flooding that the incoming reports were describing. Graham was deployed, initially as part of a rapid response team with two of his close volunteer friends, one a vet nurse, the other an Air Force Veteran. They arrived together to meet the other groups of volunteers, rural fire members, army soldiers, police, and engineers, who were also brought in to form search and recovery teams. Graham's team was tasked with checking properties before the town was 'opened up' for residents to return.

They came across an elderly lady sitting with her feet steeped in mud, unable to move but alive. They got her out. She was the last person his team found alive. As Graham and his team came in at sundown each day, they came back through the incident command tents to sign in. He saw that the volunteer peer support teams were there too. One of his mates was a peer supporter, and he was looking forward to catching up with him. He received a text saying he was thinking of him. It was good to know that they were there when he needed them. He will never forget what he saw during those

DOI: 10.4324/9781003292807-9

days: lives lost, bodies unrecognizable, a town turned into swamp, livelihoods decimated. There were rescue workers everywhere, helicopters, and army vehicles. 'All that noise and chaos… it was like a battlefield.'

Graham struggled in the aftermath of his experience. In the years following, he had dreams reliving the experience and images of the human remains he'd checked for life. He was easily triggered by remembrance broadcasts on the news each year; he would break out in sweats and had difficulties concentrating at times. Ten years later, he still doesn't like to talk about the lives lost, but he doesn't see those images in his mind anymore. Today, Graham credits the help he sought through the emergency peer-support teams to start a conversation and the healing process. They put him in touch with a psychologist whose family he had helped years before. 'Talking about it helps… It's made me stronger.' Graham had joined the state emergency services to find a sense of camaraderie and belonging. He emotively describes that he hasn't been disappointed and that the trust and companionship with his peers and the psychologist, along with the support of his family, has helped him find new meaning in his life. He treasures the time spent at soccer games with his sons, reconnected with his estranged sister after the floods, went on to start up a local men's support shed in his town, and is now a Group Leader mentoring other volunteers.

Disaster and Emergency Response Volunteer Populations – Who Are They?

Volunteer emergency and disaster workers put their hands up to band together with other workers to carry out their purpose in helping others in times of greatest need. While there are many challenges in calculating global numbers of disaster and emergency response volunteers, the figures are very large. The most recent count of all volunteers of people 15 years or older each month is 862 million across the globe, with 6.5% of this group engaged in formal volunteering via an organization or association (Millora et al., 2021). The United Nations Volunteers group categorizes this type of volunteering as Service Volunteering, which refers to responding within a formal organization to the perceived needs of a community or person (Millora et al., 2021). This type of volunteering is separated from other types of volunteering, such as spontaneous volunteering which also takes place by community members but not within a formal organizational context (Whittaker et al., 2015).

The volunteer population in disaster and emergency response is diverse. They come from all walks of life and provide their volunteer work in and around their other occupations, family lives, and community activities. They have varying demographics, levels of skills, commitments, and needs. Disaster and emergency response volunteers often addition-ally hold paid positions that range across professional roles, trades, and other volunteer roles. Britton (1991) found that volunteers within one disaster response network (e.g., ambulance, fire, state emergency services) have a tendency to hold joint positions across different emergency service organizations or to transition between the organizations as permanent volunteers. This is often seen in rural and remote locations.

Whether their other primary jobs are within or outside of disaster and emergency services, volunteers like Graham are tasked with juggling varying and conflicting job needs and responsibilities, release authoriza-tion pathways, and work commitments in order to achieve being available for deployments, often with little notice. Families of volunteers provide an essential layer of support to enable the volunteer to deploy in times of activation and are an important consideration for disaster and emergency service organizations. Disaster recovery work has a large impact on the functioning and needs of the families of volunteers (Cowlishaw et al., 2008), and they should be included along with their volunteering family member in considering easy access pathways to organisational support systems.

Compared with paid full-time staff in these organizations, volunteer arms of disaster and emergency services have different organizational structures, different day-to-day working processes, less opportunity for training, and less access to communications with supervisors and peers. Volunteers generally attend their meeting venue once a week for training, with some longer training exercises scattered throughout the year, which they balance alongside working in their other full-time or part-time jobs.

As in Graham's case, depending on the nature of rostering, many volunteers operate on an "as needs" or on-call basis, often responding operationally from their primary place of work or from home in the midst of non-related activities, with little time to engage in full psychological preparedness processes. They often respond to events within their com-munity and surrounding areas with community members in need and locations known to them and thus in a context of high emotional prox-imity, and often at a distance and isolated from the managers, controllers, or coordinators activating the response. These contextual differences can seem to the volunteer to set them apart from their full-time colleagues, and the isolation can take its toll, particularly in more mechanistic organizational volunteering models versus more organic organizational volunteering models that are relationally-based and operate more from a core expression of shared values (Rochester et al., 2010). Besides the sense of being separate or isolated from the workplace and management structures, not being present in the workplace or having regular contact with managerial and administrative staff and processes can disrupt the formation of rich and supportive bonds that volunteers highly value, par-ticularly given the dangerous nature of the volunteer work they do. The rural or remote locations of many volunteers compound these difficulties;

however, it is because they are located rurally that their positions there, where the disasters and emergencies are occurring (away from much-needed other resources), are so valuable.

There is sparse research comparing the wellbeing of career frontline workers with their counterpart volunteer cohort, and the available research represents conflicting outcomes. A study investigating mental health in volunteer firefighters in Australia uncovered a high likelihood of experiencing negative consequences from exposure to multiple high-impact events, assault, or being trapped in dangerous situations (Milligan-Saville et al., 2018). While this study did not directly compare volunteers to their paid counterparts, they did provide comparisons of their findings to a cohort of paid firefighters (Harvey et al., 2016), which were in line with the prevalence found in the volunteers. These findings vary from an American study investigating mental health differences between paid and volunteer firefighters, noting that the prevalence of mental health issues was remarkably elevated in the volunteer group and that greater structural barriers (cost and availability) to accessing mental health services statistically mediated the relationship between volunteer status and higher psychiatric symptoms (Stanley et al., 2017). Earlier work by Guo and colleagues (2004) reported higher levels of mental health issues in Chinese volunteer emergency rescue workers after helping out in the aftermath of an earthquake. One study noted the differing work contexts of Australian career and volunteer firefighter cohorts, with career firefighters having rostered shifts on duty; continual access to training and development of expertise whilst on shift; and access to colleagues before, during, and immediately after a complex job that they may wish to debrief about (Dean et al., 2003). Auxiliary firefighters (part-time volunteer firefighters) are generally on-call 24/7 and their tasks include responding to critical incident requests from the public, but unlike their professional counterparts, they have little opportunity to naturally debrief about events they attend. However, it was also noted that the group of auxiliary firefighters reported lower psychological distress than the group of career firefighters. Psychological distress reported by firefighters was seen to be influenced by attendance at duty-based traumatic events, traumatic events attended while not on duty as a firefighter, military experience, and home-related stresses. Length of service was one factor associated with higher rates of psychological distress in career firefighters, although the authors caution that other factors, including the nature of exposure to traumatic events on and off the job for that cohort, were also implicated. Cicognani and colleagues (2009) also found that volunteer emergency workers enjoyed higher levels of wellbeing and quality of life than their full-time professional counterparts. They had longer lengths of service (and expertise), higher self-efficacy, and stronger use of active coping strategies.

A problem with comparing study designs is that most research has set out to investigate psychopathology only, and few studies have investigated the broader background, motivation, and work conditions of volunteer rescue workers or even other outcomes after the experience of high-impact events, hence limiting our understanding of how to best support improved mental wellbeing in this population. Perhaps, then, a focus on why people choose to volunteer might provide a different avenue to explore potential protective mechanisms towards mental ill-health and positive post-trauma outcomes.

Bonds Forged in Fire, Flood, Storm, and Blood

> Volunteerism is a basic expression of human relationships. It is about people's need to participate in their societies and to feel that they matter to others. It is infused with values including solidarity, reciprocity, mutual trust, belonging and empowerment, all of which contribute significantly to the well-being of individuals, their communities, and societies.
>
> (U.N. Volunteers, 2011)

For disaster and emergency response volunteers, a sense of community and relationships are the primary purpose for volunteering (Beyerlein & Sikkink, 2008; Francis & Jones, 2012). In their research with Americans who volunteered for a group or organization following the September 11 terrorist attacks, Berelein & Sikkink (2008) reported that motivations to volunteer included personal feelings of responsibility to help people in need, a civic responsibility and humanitarian principle, personal or collective identification with people or the event, and connecting with affected community members as part of the broader family or tribe. Carpenter and Myers (2007), in their study of U.S. firefighters, identify that altruism and social reputation are positively correlated with volunteering. Stukas and colleagues (2016) identify altruistic values supported in benevolence (enhancing the welfare of a personal network) and universalism (enhancing the welfare of all people and of nature) are most associated with volunteer behavior and well-being, as do Francis and Jones (2012) in their research with volunteer firefighters. They identified that both new generation (aged under 35) and traditional generation (aged over 35) volunteer firefighters are equally and most highly oriented towards transcendence values of benevolence and universalism, with new generation volunteers additionally holding higher value for, and desires to increase self-efficacy in, mastering the skills that they'll be using in the course of their duties.

Rotolo and Berg (2011) highlighted the importance of social and network ties for emergency preparedness and disaster relief volunteers. They reported that almost half (46.6%) of volunteers first became involved as volunteers after being asked by someone if they would be interested in this type of task. 60% of those connections were directly made by someone in the organization. Volunteers tend to leave their volunteer roles due to not feeling valued and supported by their organizations (Fallon & Rice, 2015). Fallon and Rice (2015) compared the future turnover intention of volunteers and paid employees within an emergency service organization. They reported that perceived employee development and job satisfaction were more salient to the turnover intentions of paid employees, while support and recognition influenced job satisfaction as key motivators of volunteers' ongoing commitment to the organization.

Benevolent values, development of camaraderie, social ties, collective bonds, and friendships that last a lifetime are the primary purpose of joining a volunteer organization (Baxter-Tomkins & Wallace, 2009). In disaster, emergency service, and humanitarian aid work, collective bonds are quite literally forged in fire, flood, storm, and blood. Thus, the significance of the quality of the bonds within the organization is high, particularly with key personnel (such as the organization's managers, peer supporters, colleagues, and counsellors) whose input or lack thereof may influence the volunteer's mental health outcomes. This is illustrated by a study investigating motivation for volunteering in a group of paid and volunteer firefighters in the United States, where a strong sense for the importance of, and camaraderie with, the Chief of the fire station was noted as a main motivator to engage, and a strong sense of community and "brotherhood" provided a feeling of family and connection (Haski-Leventhal & McLeigh, 2009).

Influencing Wellbeing Pathways with Volunteers in Disaster and Emergency Response

Understanding these deeply held beliefs of volunteers; developing close, trusted, and bonded relationships within the workplace, particularly with key personnel such as the organization's managers, peer supporters, and psychologists; and creating workplace cultures of belonging are all required in order to support a volunteer's wellbeing, perhaps forming the foundations for the development of a sense of psychological safety that underlies it (Cockshaw et al., 2013; Shakespeare-Finch & Daley, 2017).

Volunteer emergency responders tend to have high levels of meaning around their work. Trust and reciprocity as aspects of the social relationship or social capital are important for the establishment of psychological security or psychological safety, which is an important foundation for overcoming barriers to accessing support, emotional expression, psychological flexibility, cognitive deliberations, and meaning-making associated with posttraumatic growth outcomes, particularly with populations like disaster and emergency response volunteers immersed in high-impact events and who hold their work with very high purpose and meaning. The importance of social capital or social cohesion (via trust, reciprocity, cooperation, and a shared sense of identification/

belonging) in promoting posttraumatic growth by enhancing the individual's psychological security has been demonstrated to be higher in cohorts who have high meaning and a sense of purpose in their jobs versus those who don't (Nie et al., 2021), as is present in volunteer disaster and emergency response workers. The development of such social capital requires mutual communication, interaction, and cooperation with the individual (Nahapiet & Ghoshal, 1998), which in emergency and disaster management organizations requires targeted strategic planning, structures, and processes in order to achieve housing-sustainable opportunities for these relational elements between volunteers, managers, colleagues, and support staff to gain depth, particularly where distance and diversions from day-to-day operations exist as they do in volunteer sectors compared with career-based operations.

It appears that whilst volunteer disaster and emergency volunteers come from all walks of life with varying demographics, levels of skills, commitments, and needs, which can make meeting those varying needs complex and highly difficult for an organization, they are mostly highly aligned with benevolent and universalist values for working for the good of their communities and deeply value a sense of belonging, camaraderie, and rich trusting and reciprocal relationships with people in their volunteer organization, which appears to influence their wellbeing and engagement – perhaps providing a light at the end of the tunnel if coordinated organizational efforts can be made with this in mind.

For Graham, the reciprocal, trusted and bonded relationships and support that he had with his family and friends, in addition to the event-focused support he received from within his relationships with his colleagues, peer supporters, and psychologist, allowed him to work through the challenging exposures to inhumane death, restricted freedoms of the elderly lady, and the gravity of the presence of the flood itself. He came to appreciate the time he had with his family and children while they were young even more, had a stronger belief in himself to take on a Group Leader position within the volunteer community, and strengthened his spiritual connection with his purpose that he was here on earth to help others and the environment. This led to him embracing the mentoring role and giving back to the land that had been decimated by taking on a revegetation project in his park ranger job. Thus we might reflect that Graham has a greater sense of coherence – the capacity or ability to comprehend, interact with, and make meaning of the world (Antonovsky, 1987) – and posttraumatic growth indicators (Tedeschi & Calhoun, 2004) following his experience of this high impact event.

Conclusion

Without disaster and emergency response volunteers, much of the disaster relief and recovery efforts coordinated by disaster management and emergency services would not be possible. Understanding their values, what brings them to volunteering, and meeting their wellbeing needs is an important endeavor for disaster and emergency response organizations.

Volunteering is steeped in deep and meaningful humanitarian purposes of altruism, civic responsibility to help communities in need, desires for belongingness, collective values, and opportunities for mastering skills to do a good job for others. If the very purpose that underlies a person's engagement with volunteering is deeply interwoven into the core beliefs about how to "be" in the world and how the world should be, the focus and strategies for supporting such volunteers need to be in alignment with these core elements.

We know from the research on PTSD, moral injury, compassion fatigue, and depression and anxiety that breaches or challenges to such beliefs are likely to create distress. Disaster and emergency management organizations need to pay attention to making appropriate types of support processes available to volunteers so that volunteers can see their early emotional distress, cognitive confusion, and upheaval in response to processing their experiences of high-impact events as normal, functional, culturally acceptable, and highly valuable experiences and pathways to growth.

It is a timely reminder for volunteer organizations to not outsource their care to other entities and processes with volunteers and to invest in the strategic planning, infrastructure development, training, and processes that see the development of wellbeing cultures capable of supporting high engagement, longevity, and wellbeing of their volunteer populations in disaster and emergence response contexts. Whilst there are many other considerations not covered in the scope of this chapter, ensuring the support of volunteers and their families through the development of these enriching cultures of belongingness, camaraderie, and pre-event development of strong, trusted, reciprocal interpersonal relationships with managers, colleagues, and support personnel may provide a significant step in allowing for the psychological safety, rest, emotional expression and meaning-making processes that lead to post-traumatic growth outcomes, engagement, and collective prosperity for the individuals, teams, families, organizations, and the communities they serve to emerge.

References

Antonovsky, A. (1987). *The salutogenic perspective: Toward a new view of health and illness.* Advances.

Baxter-Tomkins, T., & Wallace, M. (2009). Recruitment and retention of volunteers in emergency services. *Australian Journal on Volunteering, 14,* 39–49. ISSN: 1325-8362

Beyerlein, K., & Sikkink, D. (2008). Sorrow and solidarity: Why Americans volunteered for 9/11 relief efforts. *Social Problems, 55*(2), 190-215. Doi:10.1525/sp.2008.55.2.190

Britton, N. R. (1991). Permanent disaster volunteers: Where do they fit? *Nonprofit and voluntary sector quarterly, 20*(4), 395–414

Carpenter, J. P., & Myers, C.K. (2007) Why volunteer? Evidence on the role of altruism, reputation, and incentives. *The Journal of Public Economics, 94*, 11–12. doi:10.2139/ssrn.1014584

Cicognani, E., Pietrantoni, L., Palestini, L., & Prati, G. (2009). Emergency workers' quality of life: The protective role of sense of community, efficacy beliefs and coping strategies. *Social Indicators Research, 94*(3), 449. doi:10.1007/s11205-009-9441-x

Cockshaw, W. D., Shochet, I. M., & Obst, P. L. (2013). General belongingness, workplace belongingness, and depressive symptoms. *Journal of Community & Applied Social Psychology, 23*(3), 240–251. doi:10.1002/casp.2121

Cowlishaw, S., Evans, L., & McLennan, J. (2008). Families of rural volunteer firefighters. *Rural Society, 18*(1), 17–25. doi:10.5172/rsj.351.18.1.17

Dean, P. G., Gow, K. M., & Shakespeare-Finch, J. (2003). Counting the Cost: Psychological Distress in Career and Auxiliary Firefighters. *Australasian Journal of Disaster and Trauma Studies.* ISSN: 1174–4707

Fallon, B. J., & Rice, S. M. (2015). Investment in staff development within an emergency services organisation: Comparing future intention of volunteers and paid employees. *The International Journal of Human Resource Management, 26*(4), 485–500. doi:10.1080/09585192.2011.561222

Francis, J. E., & Jones, M. (2012). Emergency service volunteers: A comparison of age, motives and values. *Australian Journal of Emergency Management, 27*(4), 27–32. ISSN: 1324–1540

Guo, Y. J., Chen, C. H., Lu, M. L., Tan, H. K. L., Lee, H. W., & Wang, T. N. (2004). Posttraumatic stress disorder among professional and non-professional rescuers involved in an earthquake in Taiwan. *Psychiatry Research, 127*(1–2), 35–41. doi:10.1016/j.psychres.2004.03.009

Harvey, S. B., Milligan-Saville, J. S., Paterson, H. M., Harkness, E. L., Marsh, A. M., Dobson, M., Kemp, R., & Bryant, R. A. (2016). The mental health of fire-fighters: An examination of the impact of repeated trauma exposure. *Australian & New Zealand Journal of Psychiatry, 50*(7), 649–658. doi:10.1177/0004867415615217

Haski-Leventhal, D., & McLeigh, J. D. (2009). Firefighters volunteering beyond their duty: an essential asset in rural communities. *Journal of Rural and Community Development, 4*(2). ISSN: 1712–8277

Milligan-Saville, J., Choi, I., Deady, M., Scott, P., Tan, L., Calvo, R. A., Bryant, R. A., Glozier, N., & Harvey, S. B. (2018). The impact of trauma exposure on the development of PTSD and psychological distress in a volunteer fire service. *Psychiatry Research, 270*, 1110–1115. doi:10.1016/j.psychres.2018.06.058

Millora, C., Robinson-Pant, A., Jere, C., & Grotz, J. (2021). *2022 State of the World's Volunteerism Report: Building equal and inclusive societies*. United Nations Volunteers. https://swvr2022.unv.org/

Nahapiet, J., & Ghoshal, S. (1998). Social capital, intellectual capital, and the organizational advantage. *Academy of Management Review, 23*(2), 242–266. doi:10.5465/amr.1998.533225

Nie, T., Tian, M., & Liang, H. (2021). Relational capital and post-traumatic growth: The role of work meaning. *International Journal of Environmental Research and Public Health, 18*(14), 7362. doi:10.3390/ijerph18147362

Rochester, C., Paine, A. E., Howlett, S., & Zimmeck, M. (2010). Motivation and Recruitment: Why and how do volunteers come? In C. Rochester, A. E. Paine, S. Howlett, & M. Zimmeck (Eds.) *Volunteering and Society in the 21st Century* (pp. 119–132). Palgrave Macmillan, London. doi:10.1057/9780230279438_9

Rotolo, T., & Berg, J. A. (2011). In times of need: An examination of emergency preparedness and disaster relief service volunteers. *Nonprofit and Voluntary Sector Quarterly, 40*, 740–750. doi:10.1177/0899764010369179

Shakespeare-Finch, J., & Daley, E. (2017). Workplace belongingness, distress, and resilience in emergency service workers. *Psychological Trauma: Theory, Research, Practice, and Policy, 9*, 32–35. doi:10.1037/tra0000108

Stanley, I. H., Boffa, J. W., Hom, M. A., Kimbrel, N. A., & Joiner, T. E. (2017). Differences in psychiatric symptoms and barriers to mental health care between volunteer and career firefighters. *Psychiatry Research, 247*, 236–242. doi:10.1016/j.psychres.2016.11.037

Stukas, A. A., Snyder, M., & Clary, E. G. (2016). Understanding and encouraging volunteerism and community involvement. *The Journal of Social Psychology, 156*, 243–255. doi:10.1080/00224545.2016.1153328

Tedeschi, R. G., & Calhoun, L. G. (2004). Posttraumatic growth: conceptual foundations and empirical evidence. *Psychological Inquiry, 15*, 1–18. doi:10.1207/s15327965pli1501_01

United Nations Volunteers (2011). *The power of volunteerism*. https://www.unv.org/power-volunteerism

Whittaker, J., McLennan, B., & Handmer, J. (2015). A review of informal volunteerism in emergencies and disasters: Definition, opportunities and challenges. *International Journal of Disaster Risk Reduction, 13*, 358–368. doi:10.1016/j.ijdrr.2015.07.010

Nurses

8

Ellyse McCormick and Gillian Ray-Barruel

Kerry-Ann

> Kerry-Anne, a nurse in the renal dialysis unit, was recently involved in a workplace incident where the patient receiving hemodialysis became agitated and began shouting at her. When Kerry-Anne tried to calm him down, he began to tug at his dialysis catheter, dislodging it from his fistula. Blood began to pour over Kerry-Anne's hands as she attempted to staunch the bleeding while restraining the patient and calling for assistance.
>
> A month later, Kerry-Anne is still dreaming about the incident and feeling nauseous when she remembers the sticky wet patient's blood coating her forearms. Last night, her daughter came into the kitchen, crying and bleeding, after falling off her bike. When Kerry-Anne knelt down to soothe her daughter, she began to feel nauseous and faint. She managed to wrap paper towel around her daughter's elbow and make sure the cuts were only superficial.
>
> This morning, Kerry-Anne is feeling jittery and anxious about going to work in the dialysis unit. She dreads the thought of having an agitated patient and she is frightened about the prospect of touching another person's blood. She is thinking about transferring out of the dialysis unit to another type of ward.

Nurses account for over half the world's healthcare workforce, with 28 million nurses worldwide (World Health Organization [WHO], 2020). The COVID-19 pandemic has shone a spotlight on the vital role nurses perform and revealed the systemic cracks and crevices nurses must negotiate in their daily role. But the nursing profession has been in crisis for years, with regular reports of staff shortages, workplace violence, high turnover and absenteeism, moral and emotional distress, and high rates of burnout and depression. To combat the stressors placed on nurses, massive strategic investments in approaches to strengthen nursing education, jobs, leadership, and service delivery (WHO, 2021a) are urgently needed to improve health systems and outcomes.

DOI: 10.4324/9781003292807-10

Stress and Nurses' Mental Health

Nursing has long been recognized as a highly stressful and difficult profession. The vignette above demonstrates several common workplace triggers for nurses and the ongoing effects on the nurse if these are not properly addressed. While Kerry-Anne is fictional, this kind of scenario is all too real for nurses. In an ordinary shift, a nurse may care for patients (or visitors) who are agitated and possibly violent, and exposure to bodily fluids is a well-known occupational hazard of nursing. Experiences such as the one described may lead to an inability to mentally switch off when a shift ends; dreams about a traumatic work experience; emotions of anxiety, fear, and hypervigilance related to the workplace; and persistent dread that another traumatic event will occur at work or elsewhere.

Compounding the daily challenges of this stressful occupation is the ingrained expectation of a "duty to care," which entails altruistically putting the patient's needs before the nurse's self-interests. From the very first days of becoming a student nurse, the ethical responsibility of being the patient's advocate is reiterated and reinforced. The personal cost of such advocacy is rarely mentioned. In recent years, mindfulness and self-care have become buzzwords in popular culture, with the onus being on the individual to remember to care for themselves, or as flight attendants remind us, "put on your own oxygen mask before helping others." Self-care and self-advocacy are problematic and somewhat contradictory concepts for nurses, who juggle competing expectations and allegiance to their patients, their nursing colleagues, the organization, and the profession, as well as obligations of family, friends, and the wider community. Taking time for the self is not often a priority or even a realistic goal. Nurses cope as best they can with the competing and seemingly never-ending pressures of patient care by skipping meal breaks, foregoing toilet breaks, forgetting to keep hydrated, and staying behind after the shift to complete documentation or check in with a struggling colleague or suffering patient.

Nurses in many practice settings are routinely exposed to human suffering, disease, death, and life-threatening illness or injury. The cumulative stress of this exposure, plus unexpected workplace trauma, including physical assault and interpersonal conflicts, can severely compromise the nurse's own mental health (Stelnicki & Carleton, 2020; Stelnicki et al., 2020). The statistics for mental health problems experienced by nurses themselves are alarming. A large study of 4267 nurses in Canada identified 48% screened positive for a mental disorder (Stelnicki & Carleton, 2020). A U.S. survey of direct care nurses in three hospitals found moderate burnout rates of 54% before the COVID-19 pandemic, with high levels of emotional exhaustion and cynicism among the nurses (Kelly et al., 2021). Not surprisingly, prolonged emotional exhaustion is negatively associated with nurses' productivity and positively associated with intention to leave (Jun et al., 2021).

As a traditionally female-dominated profession, many nurses have additional caring responsibilities or study commitments when they leave work, often called the "second shift." Juggling concurrent responsibilities with staff shortages, interpersonal workplace conflicts, long shifts, and unsociable hours can lead to depression, compassion fatigue, and burnout. Furthermore, the constant stress of making difficult decisions and being unable to provide the care they know the patient needs can lead to moral distress. In a report conducted by NSI Nursing Solutions, Inc. (2022), hospitals in the U.S. were invited to participate in a survey reporting their workforce turnover data between January 2021–December 2021. In total, 272 hospitals from 32 states provided 589,901 responses; 166,087 nurses responded, revealing that nurse turnover rates in the U.S. rose by 8.4% to 27.1% in 2021, possibly related to the COVID-19 pandemic. This figure is higher than the hospital turnover rate of 25.9% in 2021 (NSI Nursing Solutions, 2022). Additionally, the average U.S. hospital turned over 95.7% of their registered nurse workforce over the past five years (NSI Nursing Solutions, 2022).

At an international convention of national nursing associations from 33 countries, 37 nurse leaders and 61 nurse representatives participated in a survey on their perceptions of nurses' mental health. Findings revealed that the majority regarded nurses' mental health as important for the provision of quality patient care, but most saw it as an individual responsibility of the nurses themselves (Wills et al., 2020). Unfortunately, this is not surprising. Although burnout is most often linked to organizational factors, strategies to reduce nurses' mental distress have largely focused on fostering individual coping skills and building resilience (Nwanya & Rowberry, 2021). While boosting individual self-efficacy skills is helpful and important, much more must be done on an organizational and governance level to reduce workplace stressors and promote nurses' work-life balance. Without targeted strategies to increase recruitment and retain existing nurses, international healthcare systems are heading for a nurse staffing crisis, particularly post-COVID-19 (Falatah, 2021).

Nurses report tension between organizational expectations, their own professional expectations of their role, and the ability to deliver care commensurate with their level of experience and patient needs. Most nurses see meaning in their work, but a lack of individual and collective agency of nurses can contribute to difficulties in comprehending organizational priorities and managing expectations (both organizational and personal) (Smeds Alenius et al., 2020). Societal expectations on nurses place an added burden. Repeated surveys have demonstrated that the public place nurses in high esteem and regard them as trustworthy and committed (Morgan, 2016). However, common stereotypes of nurses as "angels," "selfless, noble and hardworking women" (Girvin et al., 2016) bestow an onerous and inaccurate mantle on the nursing profession, reinforcing expectations that may be difficult and sometimes impossible to meet.

Nurses' strained mental health is a widespread problem that directly affects patient and organizational outcomes. A systematic review including 20 studies demonstrated an inverse relationship between nurses' burnout and patient safety and quality of care; nurses' commitment and productivity; and patient satisfaction (Jun et al., 2021). A data-linkage study in the U.S. found a significant correlation between nurses' higher burnout scores and patient surgical site and urinary tract infections; hospitals with 30% lower burnout scores had over 6200 fewer infections, with annual cost savings of $68 million (Cimiotti et al., 2012). A U.S. survey of infection prevention staff (nurses and physicians) identified that workplaces reporting higher levels of psychological safety were also more likely to implement evidence-based infection practices, such as urinary catheter stop-orders or sedation vacations for ventilated patients (Greene et al., 2020).

The ethos of healthcare is to "first do no harm." When patient harm occurs, nurses and other healthcare workers may question how their own actions might have led to the event, even if they did everything by the book. So-called "second victims" are frontline workers who have been emotionally traumatized by unanticipated, adverse patient events, particularly if they feel personally responsible for the event (Dekker, 2013; Draus et al., 2022; Wu, 2000). When a healthcare worker perceives their actions may have caused direct or indirect, actual or potential harm to a patient in their care, it can lead to feelings of guilt and moral distress. Staff shortages and resource constraints amplify moral distress by making it impossible for staff to provide the care they believe the patient needs.

The COVID-19 Pandemic

The COVID-19 pandemic created extra strain on the chronically underfunded and already vulnerable healthcare workforce. In the early days of the pandemic, nurses were at the forefront of navigating unchartered patient care territory while also adjusting to the changing world around them. Suddenly, personal protective equipment (PPE) shortages were common, and transmission of the illness and mortality rate was unknown. The media was filled with horror stories of people saying goodbye to loved ones via video call and dying alone. Ethical challenges arose as resource shortages meant people were prioritized for ventilators depending on their perceived quality of life: a triage decision with enormous moral implications (Ferorelli et al., 2020). Staff were reusing masks and other PPE due to a worldwide shortage, all the while not knowing what impact COVID-19 would have in the long term. Before the availability of coronavirus vaccines, healthcare professionals were contracting COVID-19 and still having to go to work because there weren't enough staff to care for the increasing volume of patients. In September 2021, the World Health Organization released a report confirming that 6643 healthcare workers had died in the first 15 months of the pandemic but estimating the real number to be between 80,000–160,000 deaths, based on population estimates (WHO, 2021b). There was also the added fear and risk of bringing the virus home and infecting their family members and knowing that going to work meant added stress for their families. Viewing television or social media became too traumatic at times, as nurses worldwide counted down the days until these images became reality in their own workplace. Widely hailed by many as "heroes" or "angels" for their seemingly superhuman commitment to providing patient care during the pandemic, globally nurses also have had to shoulder the burden of community frustration, fear, and vaccine hesitancy, often while caring for their own families, home-schooling children, and performing caring duties for elderly and disabled relatives.

The COVID-19 pandemic drastically challenged the way nurses provide meaningful and holistic care to patients, contributing to widespread moral distress, depression, anxiety, burnout, vicarious trauma, and posttraumatic stress disorder (PTSD) among the profession. The pandemic greatly exacerbated the stressors nurses experience in the workplace, with several recent workforce surveys revealing the extent of nurses experiencing depression, anxiety, and burnout (Aggar et al., 2022; Cai et al., 2020; Denning et al., 2021; Ohue et al., 2021; Pachi et al., 2022; Schierberl Scherr et al., 2021; Smallwood, Karimi, et al., 2021); moral distress (Smallwood et al., 2021); prolonged workplace-induced trauma (Jiang et al., 2022; Smallwood, Pascoe, et al., 2021; Zeiher et al., 2022); and wanting to leave the profession (Mai et al., 2022; Ohue et al., 2021; Zeiher et al., 2022). A survey in Germany identified fear of contracting infection, insufficient supplies of PPE, and feeling unequipped to deal with severely ill patients as contributing to burnout in 47% of nurse respondents, with 20% planning to leave nursing after the pandemic (Mai et al., 2022). In a large survey of Australian healthcare workers (39% nurses), respondents identified resource scarcity (58%); wearing PPE (32%); excluding families from visiting the patients (60%); and fear of letting down co-workers (55%) as major contributors to moral distress, which was associated with increased risk of anxiety, depression, burnout, and PTSD (Smallwood, Pascoe, et al., 2021).

Conversely, other surveys have identified posttraumatic growth among nurses following COVID-19, correlating with higher self-efficacy and social support (Li et al., 2022; Mo et al., 2022; Peng et al., 2021; Yeung et al., 2022; Zhang et al., 2021), professional identity (Mo et al., 2022), and feeling appreciated by the community (Smallwood, Pascoe, et al., 2021). Interviews with U.S. nurses working on the frontline throughout the pandemic reported the importance of peer support from colleagues, but disappointment in the perceived chaotic response from hospital management to requests for more PPE and other resources, and a corresponding sense of their own disposability from the organizational perspective (Jun & Rosemberg, 2021).

From stress, posttraumatic growth can occur and two years on, healthcare and the world have transitioned to living with COVID-19 with vaccines now widely available (Cui et al., 2021). One qualitative study of nurses working in the COVID-19 isolation ward during the pandemic highlighted initial negative emotions such as anxiety, fear of the unknown, and fear of the impact on their families (Sun et al., 2020). The nurses then engaged in coping mechanisms such as distraction, humor, isolation, journaling, meditation, mindfulness, venting, and exercise as useful methods to adapt to their new reality. The nurses also spoke of colleague support as good stress relief and described how the challenges they worked through together enhanced team cohesion. Other positive coping strategies included maintaining a calm attitude, using medical knowledge to analyze the situation, and taking the initiative to encourage themselves and find solutions. This process led to increased gratitude for their own health, their future, and for social support including friends/family and colleagues. The nurses also expressed a deeper appreciation for their professional identity and the importance of the nursing profession (Sun et al., 2020).

Posttraumatic Growth

Nurses are versatile, highly capable workers, and the profession of nursing offers an enormous range of career options, many with flexible schedules, travel opportunities, and decent pay. Work satisfaction is often high, particularly in workplaces with strong support from management and co-workers. Nurses experience great satisfaction from helping patients to get better or to ease their suffering. Many describe the role of nursing as a privilege, being there for patients and families at a time when they are most vulnerable and being able to offer practical or emotional support. Nurses are witnesses to the most fundamental and emotional human aspects of life, from birth to sickness and death. Highly charged working environments such as the emergency department or critical care units create an adrenaline rush and the satisfaction that comes from applying one's knowledge and skills to save lives. Finding meaning in work has a protective effect against burnout and stress (Hamama-Raz et al., 2021).

Self-esteem and ability to deal with stress are influenced by a sense of comprehensibility, manageability, and meaningfulness (Kupcewicz, 2022), otherwise termed a sense of coherence. Studies have found that nurses with a stronger sense of coherence use more adaptive coping strategies to deal with stress and report lower levels of alcohol and drug use (Betke et al., 2021) and report less depression, burnout, and job dissatisfaction (Masanotti et al., 2020). A stronger sense of coherence can partially mediate depression and burnout among nurses (Mai et al., 2022; Pachi et al., 2022). In a Portuguese survey of 400 nurses, attribution of social worth to the nursing role was associated with greater wellbeing and less burnout (Santos et al., 2020).

Mindfulness-based stress reduction strategies have increased in popularity over the last decade with some evidence of their effectiveness for healthcare workers in general (Gilmartin et al., 2017). Popular strategies to boost nurses' wellbeing include meditation apps and encouraging text-messages (Kelly, Schaeffer, et al., 2021). Nominal group discussions with emergency department nurses in Australia elicited wellness strategies that the nurses themselves believed would be helpful; strategies included mobile/web-based applications, yoga, social activities, team-building activities, group counselling sessions, and debriefing (Elder et al., 2021). However, most intervention studies examining wellness strategies for nurses have had small sample sizes with limited longitudinal follow-up, and therefore more research is needed (Elder et al., 2020; Xu et al., 2020).

Psychological guidance and support programs can promote nurses' posttraumatic growth by teaching strategies for deliberate rumination following traumatic events. Emergency department and critical care nurses repeatedly encounter trauma, violence, and unexpected death in the workplace. Positive self-compassion was found to be the biggest predictor of posttraumatic growth in one study of Chinese nurses (Chang et al., 2021). Deliberate rumination, mature age, wisdom, and self-compassion have been linked to posttraumatic growth in intensive care nurses (Chang et al., 2021). A resilience and posttraumatic growth intervention program conducted in Victoria, Australia proved successful in improving wellbeing among mental health nurses. This novel intervention delivered by trained facilitators should be trialed in other nursing departments to assist with managing the impacts of occupational stress (Foster et al., 2018).

What do Nurses need to Thrive at Work?

Organizations, such as hospitals, have a responsibility to provide a safe workplace, yet failed "zero tolerance for violence" policies still exist and staff still report frequent exposure to occupational violence as a cause of stress (Greenslade et al., 2020). Patients with acute or chronic alterations in mental state resulting from electrolyte imbalances, adverse medication responses, alcohol withdrawal, illicit substances, cognitive decline and delirium, and acute stress reactions are all common scenarios in healthcare settings that can lead to agitation and violence against staff, and while occupational violence is not always predictable, it does entail consequences, such as in the vignette described above. One study concluded that the mental health of nurses deteriorates with increased exposure to workplace violence (Fan et al., 2021). Organizations have a responsibility to protect nurses from workplace violence, support nurses when it does occur, and provide a safe working environment.

The nursing profession has been recognized as one of the highest stress careers (Goddard et al., 2021). Heavy workloads/poor skill mix, inability to provide optimal care, and overcrowding have been cited as highly stressful in emergency department nurses and doctors (Crilly et al., 2019; Greenslade et al., 2020; McCormick et al., 2023). Nursing will always be a profession that requires intentional effort to mitigate, respond to, support, and encourage opportunities for growth following incidents affecting wellbeing. These efforts should be a shared responsibility between individuals and the organization (Shanafelt & Noseworthy, 2016), with individuals responsible for seeking help when needed, engaging in adaptive and positive coping strategies, and taking regular earned recreational leave. Organizations are responsible for reducing foreseeable exposure to stress, providing adequate resourcing and staffing, equal opportunity, fairness at work, building a supportive and psychologically safe working environment, and employing and fostering transformative leaders.

A report undertaken by The King's Fund in the U.K. during 2020 identified three core work needs for nurses and midwives to thrive at work (West et al., 2020). These were a sense of belonging, autonomy, and finding meaning in work as ways to mitigate workplace stress. Firstly, nurses need to feel a sense of belonging to a team at work. Secondly, nurses need a sense of autonomy over their work life, work conditions, and schedules. Thirdly, nurses need to feel like their work is meaningful and that their contribution is valued and in alignment with individual values. The Kings Fund report outlined eight key recommendations for transforming the working lives of nurses and midwives to enhance workforce sustainability. These include:

Key recommendation 1: Authority, empowerment and influence

Introduce mechanisms for nursing and midwifery staff to shape the cultures and processes of their organizations and influence decisions about how care is structured and delivered.

Key recommendation 2: Justice and fairness

Nurture and sustain just, fair and psychologically safe cultures and ensure equity, proactive and positive approaches to diversity and universal inclusion.

Key recommendation 3: Work conditions and working schedules

Introduce minimum standards for facilities and working conditions for nursing and midwifery staff in all health and care organizations.

Key recommendation 4: Teamworking

Develop and support effective multidisciplinary teamworking for all nursing and midwifery staff across health and care services.

Key recommendation 5: Culture and leadership

Ensure health and care environments have compassionate leadership and nurturing cultures that enable both care and staff support to be high-quality, continually improving and compassionate.

Key recommendation 6: Workload

Tackle chronic excessive work demands in nursing and midwifery, which exceed the capacity of nurses and midwives to sustainably lead and deliver safe, high-quality care and which damage their health and wellbeing.

Key recommendation 7: Management and supervision

Ensure all nursing and midwifery staff have the effective support, professional reflection, mentorship and supervision needed to thrive in their roles.

Key recommendation 8: Learning, education and development

Ensure the right systems, frameworks and processes are in place for nurses' and midwives' learning, education and development throughout their careers. These must also promote fair and equitable outcomes.

(West et al. 2020, pp. 121–126)

A 2021 McKinsey & Company survey of 395 frontline nurses in the U.S. highlighted the importance of open communication, recognition, flexibility, and opportunity for nursing input into decision-making (Berlin et al., 2021). Nurses understandably expect to be safe at work, and they expect employers to provide safety equipment (including PPE); compensation for added risks (such as during the pandemic); and mental health and wellbeing resources (Berlin et al., 2021). Senior management should make concerted efforts to understand what their nurses need, address their biggest concerns, and advocate for nurses at an organizational level to challenge the status quo. By providing optimal working conditions for thriving, nurses can focus on providing quality care to patients while having time for strengthening protective factors to buffer their own professional wellbeing.

Creating a Psychologically-safe Work Environment

Developing and maintaining a psychologically safe working environment is essential for patient safety and staff retention. Stronger perceptions of management support and fairness increase nurses' trust in their supervisor and commitment to their workplace (Babamiri et al., 2021). Organizational context and manager support can have follow-on effects on the quality of patient care delivery. A questionnaire study of nurses and patients in Italy confirmed that when nurses were satisfied with the leadership, they experienced less burnout, and patients' perceptions of the nursing care were higher (Zaghini et al., 2020). Hospitals with a less-supportive culture have higher staff turnover and staff sick leave, and a higher rate of patient safety incidents, such as falls and medication errors (Dugan et al., 1996). Programs such as Magnet (American Nurses

Credentialling Center) recognize hospitals that implement strategies to retain nurses, including better nurse-patient ratios, opportunities for career advancement, and participation in nursing research, among others (Kutney-Lee et al., 2016; Kutney-Lee et al., 2015; Stone et al., 2019). Organizations that offer training and career opportunities for nurses are also reported to improve nurses' sense of coherence (Mai et al., 2022).

Incivility in the workplace can increase emotional exhaustion, while daily social support at work has shown strong benefits to nurses' vitality and wellbeing in a study in Spain (Carmona-Cobo & Lopez-Zafra, 2021). A study of nurses in China found social support in the workplace to increase nurses' sense of coherence by 58% (Zhan et al., 2020). Managers could invest in staff social activities, such as barbecue lunches or cupcake days, or encourage out-of-hours staff gatherings (for example, family picnics or movie nights) to improve workplace cohesion and job satisfaction.

Nurses often experience vicarious trauma while caring for victims of trauma, particularly when they feel ill-prepared to cope with the enormity of the situation. With the frequent exposure of nurses to trauma in the workplace and the ongoing physical and emotional effects, nursing undergraduate and graduate programs should provide trauma-informed training to prepare nurses for clinical practice (Wheeler & Phillips, 2021). Without specific and holistic education in understanding trauma – its causes, contributing factors and sequelae – and training in the skills to foster resilience and self-efficacy, nurses cannot be expected to continue to perform in highly stressful situations without suffering consequences to their own mental health, including depression, anxiety, compassion fatigue, moral distress, burnout, and PTSD (Wheeler & Phillips, 2021).

Recognizing nurses are at risk of organizational stress-induced mental health problems is an important step to healing in the profession. Reducing stigma about seeking help is also critical and can be achieved with open dialogue about the importance of psychological and physical wellbeing, making it 'okay to ask for help'. Organizations should provide all employees with information about available and accessible resources for supporting mental health and wellbeing (Berlin et al., 2021). Bolstering employee wellbeing and psychological safety is in the organization's best interests as well, with reduced staff turnover and absenteeism, and improved patient safety outcomes.

Summary

Kerry-Anne spoke to her Nurse Manager about the traumatic incident with the hemodialysis patient. The Nurse Manager listened to her story, then referred Kerry-Anne to the staff employee assistance program and arranged a meeting with the dialysis nursing team to explore the issue of workplace violence and discuss possible solutions. The Nurse Manager also requested the organizational psychologist to attend the meeting and provide support and possible solutions. The nurses decided to create a workplace covenant to state violence would not be accepted. They created posters to display in the patient areas and the staff tearoom, and they reminded patients on arrival to the unit that respect towards staff was non-negotiable. Duress alarms were installed in the dialysis unit, and a buddy system was implemented so that no nurse would ever be left alone with a patient in the unit. A quiet space adjacent to the staff tearoom was decorated with colorful cushions and soft lighting to provide a space for reflection or meditation for the staff. Her nursing colleagues decided to hold a morning tea for Kerry-Anne to show her how much they appreciated her contribution to the team and how sorry they would be if she transferred to another unit. Kerry-Anne felt moved and supported by the efforts of her manager and co-workers, and she decided to stay in the unit.

Working in the nursing profession is like going camping in the wild and being exposed to the elements. There is a gazebo keeping everyone warm and dry while waiting for the storm that is coming. It's the team who spends time securing the gazebo so that it's strong enough to weather the storm, and each rope is critical for survival. If one rope is loose, the rest suffer, and the rain gets in. These ropes are compassionate, empowering, and trusting leadership; the ability to provide meaningful and optimal care to patients; social connection at work between colleagues, with humor and shared experiences; a sense of purpose that everyone is in it together whether celebrating the wins or mourning the losses; the skills and resources to do quality work; ongoing education and learning; a supportive growth culture to foster success; flexible rostering; and enough downtime for self-care in between the storms, both at work and at home (however that looks for each individual). Nurses need time and space between storms to re-anchor, process, and grow. It is a shared responsibility between the organization and the individual to hammer the pegs back in together so they can weather the next storm. This chapter has argued that organizational imperatives and care for nurses are not competing priorities but are complementary. A salutogenic approach to workplace wellbeing offers nurses the opportunity to grow and reshape their responses to traumatic events, constructively encouraging growth and creating a deeply resilient workforce that can provide more empathic care to the patients and to each other.

References

Aggar, C., Samios, C., Penman, O., Whiteing, N., Massey, D., Rafferty, R., Bowen, K., & Stephens, A. (2022). The impact of COVID-19 pandemic-related stress experienced by Australian nurses. *International Journal of Mental Health Nursing, 31*, 91–103. doi:10.1111/inm.12938

Babamiri, M., Abdi, Z., & Noori, N. (2021). Investigating the factors that influence Iranian nurses' workplace happiness. *Nursing Management (Harrow)*, *28*, 21–28. doi:10.7748/nm.2021.e1972

Berlin, G., Lapointe, M., Murphy, M., & Viscardi, M. (2021). *Nursing in 2021: Retaining the healthcare workforce when we need it most*. Retrieved from: https://www.mckinsey.com/industries/healthcare-systems-and-services/our-insights/nursing-in-2021-retaining-the-healthc are-workforce-when-we-need-it-most

Betke, K., Basińska, M. A., & Andruszkiewicz, A. (2021). Sense of coherence and strategies for coping with stress among nurses. *BMC Nursing*, *20*, 107. doi:10.1186/s12912-021-00631-1

Cai, Z., Cui, Q., Liu, Z., Li, J., Gong, X., Liu, J., Wan, Z., Yuan, X., Li, X., Chen, C., & Wang, G. (2020). Nurses endured high risks of psychological problems under the epidemic of COVID-19 in a longitudinal study in Wuhan China. *Journal of Psychiatric Research*, *131*, 132–137. doi:10.1016/j.jpsychires.2020.09.007

Carmona-Cobo, I., & Lopez-Zafra, E. (2021). Hospital nurses experiencing day-to-day workplace incivility: A diary study on the benefits of daily social support. *Journal of Nursing Management*, *30*, 1557–1589. doi:10.1111/jonm.13510

Chang, A. K., Yoon, H., & Jang, J. H. (2021). Predictors of posttraumatic growth of intensive care unit nurses in Korea. *Japan Journal of Nursing Science*, *18*, e12427. doi:10.1111/jjns.12427

Cimiotti, J. P., Aiken, L. H., Sloane, D. M., & Wu, E. S. (2012). Nurse staffing, burnout, and health care-associated infection. *American Journal of Infection Control*, *40*, 486–490. doi:10.1016/j.ajic.2012.02.029

Crilly, J., Greenslade, J. H., Johnston, A., Carlstrom, E., Thom, O., Abraham, L., Mills, D., & Wallis, M. (2019). Staff perceptions of the emergency department working environment: An international cross-sectional survey. *Emergency Medicine Australasia*, *31*, 1082–1091. doi:10.1111/1742-6723.13325

Cui, P. P., Wang, P. P., Wang, K., Ping, Z., Wang, P., & Chen, C. (2021). Post-traumatic growth and influencing factors among frontline nurses fighting against COVID-19. *Occupational and Environmental Medicine*, *78*, 129–135. doi:10.1136/oemed-2020-106540

Dekker, S. (2013). *Second Victim: Error, Guilt, Ttrauma, and Resilience*. Boca Raton: CRC Press, Taylor & Francis Group

Denning, M., Goh, E. T., Tan, B., Kanneganti, A., Almonte, M., Scott, A., Martin, G., Clarke, J., Sounerajah, V., Markar, S., Przybylowicz, J., Chan, Y. H., Sia, C., Chua, Y., Sim, K., Lim, L., Tan, L., Tan, M., Sharma, V., Ooi, S., Beatty, J. W., Flott, K., mason, S., Chidambaram, S., Yalamanchili, S., Zbikowska, G., Fedorowski, J., Dykowska, G., Wells, M., Purkayastha, S., & Kinross, J. (2021). Determinants of burnout and other aspects of psychological well-being in healthcare workers during the Covid-19 pandemic: A multinational cross-sectional study. *PLoS One*, *16*, e0238666. doi:10.1371/journal.pone.0238666

Draus, C., Mianecki, T. B., Musgrove, H., Bastien, D. J., Greggs, D., Halash, C., Larry-Osman Bellamy, C., Lewis, A., & Mackenzie, W. (2022). Perceptions of nurses who are second victims in a hospital setting. *Journal of Nursing Care Quality*, 37, 110–116. doi:10.1097/ncq.0000000000000603

Dugan, J., Lauer, E., Bouquot, Z., Dutro, B. K., Smith, M., & Widmeyer, G. (1996). Stressful nurses: The effect on patient outcomes. *Journal of Nursing Care Quality*, 10, 46–58. Retrieved from: https://www.ncbi.nlm.nih.gov/pubmed/8634470

Elder, E., Johnston, A. N., Byrne, J. H., Wallis, M., & Crilly, J. (2021). Core components of a staff wellness strategy in emergency departments: A clinician-informed nominal group study. *Emergency Medicine Australasia*, 33, 25–33. doi:10.1111/1742-6723.13561

Elder, E., Johnston, A. N., Wallis, M., & Crilly, J. (2020). Work-based strategies/interventions to ameliorate stressors and foster coping for clinical staff working in emergency departments: a scoping review of the literature. *Australasian Emergency Care*, 23, 181–192. doi:10.1016/j.auec.2020.02.002

Falatah, R. (2021). The impact of the coronavirus disease (COVID-19) pandemic on nurses' turnover intention: An integrative review. *Nursing Reports*, 11, 787–810. doi:10.3390/nursrep11040075

Fan, S., An, W., Zeng, L., Liu, J., Tang, S., Chen, J., & Huang, H. (2021). Rethinking "zero tolerance": A moderated mediation model of mental resilience and coping strategies in workplace violence and nurses' mental health. *Journal of Nursing Scholarship*, 54, 501–512. doi:10.1111/jnu.12753

Ferorelli, D., Mandarelli, G., & Solarino, B. (2020). Ethical challenges in health care policy during COVID-19 pandemic in Italy. *Medicina (Kaunas, Lithuania)*, 56, 691. doi:10.3390/medicina56120691

Foster, K., Shochet, I., Wurfl, A., Roche, M., Maybery, D., Shakespeare-Finch, J., & Furness, T. (2018). On PAR: A feasibility study of the Promoting Adult Resilience programme with mental health nurses. *International Journal of Mental Health Nursing*, 27, 1470–1480. doi:10.1111/inm.12447

Gilmartin, H., Goyal, A., Hamati, M. C., Mann, J., Saint, S., & Chopra, V. (2017). Brief mindfulness practices for healthcare providers: A systematic literature review. *American Journal of Medicine*, 130, 1219 e1211–1219 e1217. doi:10.1016/j.amjmed.2017.05.041

Girvin, J., Jackson, D., & Hutchinson, M. (2016). Contemporary public perceptions of nursing: A systematic review and narrative synthesis of the international research evidence. *Journal of Nursing Management*, 24, 994–1006. doi:10.1111/jonm.12413

Goddard, A., Jones, R. W., Esposito, D., & Janicek, E. (2021). Trauma informed education in nursing: A call for action. *Nurse Education Today*, 101, 104880. doi:10.1016/j.nedt.2021.104880

Greene, M. T., Gilmartin, H. M., & Saint, S. (2020). Psychological safety and infection prevention practices: Results from a national survey. *American Journal of Infection Control, 48*, 2–6. doi:10.1016/j.ajic.2019.09.027

Greenslade, J. H., Wallis, M., Johnston, A. N. B., Carlstrom, E., Wilhelms, D. B., & Crilly, J. (2020). Key occupational stressors in the ED: An international comparison. *Emergency Medicine Journal, 37*, 106–111. doi:10.1136/emermed-2018-208390

Hamama-Raz, Y., Hamama, L., Pat-Horenczyk, R., Stokar, Y. N., Zilberstein, T., & Bron-Harlev, E. (2021). Posttraumatic growth and burnout in pediatric nurses: The mediating role of secondary traumatization and the moderating role of meaning in work. *Stress and Health, 37*, 442–453. doi:10.1002/smi.3007

Jiang, H., Huang, N., Tian, W., Shi, S., Yang, G., & Pu, H. (2022). Factors associated with post-traumatic stress disorder among nurses during COVID-19. *Frontiers in Psychology, 13*, 745158. doi:10.3389/fpsyg.2022.745158

Jun, J., Ojemeni, M. M., Kalamani, R., Tong, J., & Crecelius, M. L. (2021). Relationship between nurse burnout, patient and organizational outcomes: Systematic review. *International Journal of Nursing Studies, 119*, 103933. doi:10.1016/j.ijnurstu.2021.103933

Jun, J., & Rosemberg, M. S. (2021). I am a nurse, not a martyr: Qualitative investigation of nurses' experiences during onset of the coronavirus pandemic. *Policy, Politics & Nursing Practice, 23*, 48–55. doi:10.1177/15271544211054435

Kelly, L. A., Gee, P. M., & Butler, R. J. (2021). Impact of nurse burnout on organizational and position turnover. *Nursing Outlook, 69*, 96–102. doi:10.1016/j.outlook.2020.06.008

Kelly, L. A., Schaeffer, R., Roe, S., & Buchda, V. L. (2021). Using text messages to support nurse well-being. *Nursing Administration Quarterly, 45*, 338–345. doi:10.1097/NAQ.0000000000000490

Kupcewicz, E. (2022). Global self-esteem and stress intensity in a group of polish nurses—a mediatory role of a sense of coherence. *International Journal of Environmental Research and Public Health, 19*, 975. doi:10.3390/ijerph19020975

Kutney-Lee, A., Germack, H., Hatfield, L., Kelly, S., Maguire, P., Dierkes, A., Del Guidice, M., & Aiken, L. H. (2016). Nurse engagement in shared governance and patient and nurse outcomes. *Journal of Nursing Administration, 46*, 605–612. doi:10.1097/nna.0000000000000412

Kutney-Lee, A., Stimpfel, A. W., Sloane, D. M., Cimiotti, J. P., Quinn, L. W., & Aiken, L. H. (2015). Changes in patient and nurse outcomes associated with Magnet hospital recognition. *Medical Care, 53*, 550–557. doi:10.1097/mlr.0000000000000355

Li, L., Mao, M., Wang, S., Yin, R., Yan, H. O., Jin, Y., & Cheng, Y. (2022). Posttraumatic growth in Chinese nurses and general public during the COVID-19 outbreak. *Psychology, Health & Medicine, 27*, 301–311. doi:10.1080/13548506.2021.1897148

Mai, T., Todisco, L., Schilder, M., Franke, V., & Ristau, J. (2022). The situation of nurses in hospitals during the second wave of the COVID-19 pandemic: An online survey. *Pflege, 35*, 104–113. doi:10.1024/1012-5302/a000846

Masanotti, G. M., Paolucci, S., Abbafati, E., Serratore, C., & Caricato, M. (2020). Sense of coherence in nurses: A systematic review. *International Journal of Environmental Research and Public Health, 17*, 1861. doi:10.3390/ijerph17061861

McCormick, E., Devine, S., Crilly, J., Brough, P., & Greenslade, J. (2023). Measuring occupational stress in emergency departments. *Emergency Medicine Australasia, 35*, 234–241. doi: 10.1111/1742-6723.14101

Mo, Y., Tao, P., Liu, G., Chen, L., Li, G., Lu, S., Zhang, G., Liang, R., & Huang, H. (2022). Post-traumatic growth of nurses who faced the COVID-19 epidemic and its correlation with professional self-identity and social support. *Frontiers in Psychiatry, 12*. doi:10.3389/fpsyt.2021.562938

Morgan, R. (2016). Roy Morgan image of professions survey 2016: Nurses still most highly regarded followed by Doctors, Pharmacists and Engineers. Retrieved from Melbourne, Victoria: http://www.roymorgan.com/findings/6797-image-of-professions-2016-201605110031

NSI Nursing Solutions, Inc. (2022). 2022 NSI national health care retention & RN staffing report. Retrieved from https://www.nsinursingsolutions.com/Documents/Library/NSI_National_Health_Care_Retention_Report.pdf

Nwanya, M., & Rowberry, D. (2021). The importance of understanding burnout: An oncology nurse perspective. *British Journal of Nursing, 30*, S8–S14. doi:10.12968/bjon.2021.30.10.S8

Ohue, T., Togo, E., Ohue, Y., & Mitoku, K. (2021). Mental health of nurses involved with COVID-19 patients in Japan, intention to resign, and influencing factors. *Medicine (Baltimore), 100*, e26828. doi:10.1097/MD.0000000000026828

Pachi, A., Sikaras, C., Ilias, I., Panagiotou, A., Zyga, S., Tsironi, M., Baras, S., Tsitrouli, L. A., & Tselebis, A. (2022). Burnout, depression and sense of coherence in nurses during the pandemic crisis. *Healthcare (Basel), 10*, 134. doi:10.3390/healthcare10010134

Peng, X., Zhao, H. Z., Yang, Y., Rao, Z. L., Hu, D. Y., & He, Q. (2021). Post-traumatic growth level and its influencing factors among frontline nurses during the COVID-19 pandemic. *Frontiers in Psychiatry, 12*, 632360. doi:10.3389/fpsyt.2021.632360

Santos, A., Chambel, M. J., & Castanheira, F. (2020). Wellbeing among hospital nurses: A cross-sectional study of the contributions of relational job characteristics. *International Journal of Nursing Studies, 105*, 103438. doi:10.1016/j.ijnurstu.2019.103438

Schierberl Scherr, A. E., Ayotte, B. J., & Kellogg, M. B. (2021). Moderating roles of resilience and social support on psychiatric and practice outcomes in nurses working during the COVID-19 pandemic. *SAGE Open Nursing, 7.* doi:10.1177/23779608211024213

Shanafelt, T. D., & Noseworthy, J. H. (2016). Executive leadership and physician well-being. *Mayo Clinic Proceedings, 92,* 129–146. doi:10.1016/j.mayocp.2016.10.004

Smallwood, N., Karimi, L., Bismark, M., Putland, M., Johnson, D., Dharmage, S. C., &Willis, K. (2021). High levels of psychosocial distress among Australian frontline healthcare workers during the COVID-19 pandemic: A cross-sectional survey. *General Psychiatry, 34,* e100577. doi:10.1136/gpsych-2021-100577

Smallwood, N., Pascoe, A., Karimi, L., & Willis, K. (2021). Moral distress and perceived community views are associated with mental health symptoms in frontline health workers during the COVID-19 pandemic. *International Journal of Environmental Research and Public Health, 18,* 8723. doi:10.3390/ijerph18168723

Smeds Alenius, L., Lindqvist, R., Ball, J. E., Sharp, L., Lindqvist, O., & Tishelman, C. (2020). Between a rock and a hard place: Registered nurses' accounts of their work situation in cancer care in Swedish acute care hospitals. *European Journal of Oncology Nursing, 47,* 101778. doi:10.1016/j.ejon.2020.101778

Stelnicki, A. M., & Carleton, R. N. (2020). Mental disorder symptoms among nurses in Canada. *Canadian Journal of Nursing Research, 53,* 264–276. doi:10.1177/0844562120961894

Stelnicki, A. M., Jamshidi, L., Ricciardelli, R., & Carleton, R. N. (2020). Exposures to potentially psychologically traumatic events among nurses in Canada. *Canadian Journal of Nursing Research, 53,* 277–291. doi:10.1177/0844562120961988

Stone, L., Arneil, M., Coventry, L., Casey, V., Moss, S., Cavadino, A., Laing, B., & McCarthy, A. L. (2019). Benchmarking nurse outcomes in Australian Magnet® hospitals: Cross-sectional survey. *BMC Nursing, 18,* 62. doi:10.1186/s12912-019-0383-6

Sun, N., Wei, L., Shi, S., Jiao, D., Song, R., Ma, L., Wang. H., Wang, C., Wang, Z., You, Y., Liu, S., & Wang, H. (2020). A qualitative study on the psychological experience of caregivers of COVID-19 patients. *American Journal of Infection Control, 48,* 592–598. doi:10.1016/j.ajic.2020.03.018

West, M., Bailey, S., & Williams, E. (2020). The courage of compassion: Supporting nurses and midwives to deliver high-quality care. Retrieved from https://www.kingsfund.org.uk/sites/default/files/2020-09/The%20courage%20of%20compassion%20full%20report_0.pdf

Wheeler, K., & Phillips, K. E. (2021). The development of trauma and resilience competencies for nursing education. *Journal of the American Psychiatric Nurses Association, 27,* 322–333. doi:10.1177/1078390319878779

Wills, J., Hancock, C., & Nuttall, M. (2020). The health of the nursing workforce. A survey of National Nurse Associations. *International Nursing Review, 67,* 294–299. doi:10.1111/inr.12586

World Health Organization (WHO) (2020). State of the world's nursing 2020: Investing in education, jobs and leadership. Retrieved from Geneva: https://apps.who.int/iris/handle/10665/331677

World Health Organization (WHO) (2021a). *Global strategic directions for nursing and midwifery 2021–2025.* Retrieved from Geneva: https://apps.who.int/iris/handle/10665/344562

World Health Organization (WHO) (2021b). *The impact of COVID-19 on health and care workers: A closer look at deaths. Health Workforce Department Working paper 1.* Retrieved from Geneva: https://apps.who.int/iris/handle/10665/345300

Wu, A. W. (2000). Medical error: The second victim. *British Medical Journal, 320,* 726–727. doi:10.1136/bmj.320.7237.726 %J BMJ

Xu, H. G., Kynoch, K., Tuckett, A., & Eley, R. (2020). Effectiveness of interventions to reduce emergency department staff occupational stress and/or burnout: a systematic review. *JBI Evid Synth, 18,* 1156–1188. doi:10.11124/JBISRIR-D-19-00252

Yeung, N. C., Wong, E. L., Cheung, A. W., Leung, C. S., Yeoh, E. K., & Wong, S. Y. (2022). Finding the positives from the COVID-19 pandemic: Factors associated with posttraumatic growth among nurses in Hong Kong. *European Journal of Psychotraumatology, 13,* 2005346. doi:10.1080/20008198.2021.2005346

Zaghini, F., Fiorini, J., Piredda, M., Fida, R., & Sili, A. (2020). The relationship between nurse managers' leadership style and patients' perception of the quality of the care provided by nurses: Cross sectional survey. *International Journal of Nursing Studies, 101,* 103446. doi:10.1016/j.ijnurstu.2019.103446

Zeiher, W., Sego, E., Trimmer, D., & Bowers, C. (2022). Posttraumatic stress disorder in nurses during a pandemic: Implications for nurse leaders. *Journal of Nursing Administration, 52,* E3–E8. doi:10.1097/NNA.0000000000001112

Zhan, T., Li, H., & Ding, X. (2020). Can social support enhance sense of coherence and perceived professional benefits among Chinese registered nurses? A mediation model. *Journal of Nursing Management, 28,* 488–494. doi:10.1111/jonm.12931

Zhang, X. T., Shi, S. S., Qin Ren, Y., & Wang, L. (2021). The traumatic experience of clinical nurses during the COVID-19 pandemic: Which factors are related to post-traumatic growth? *Risk Management and Healthcare Policy, 14,* 2145–2151. doi:10.2147/RMHP.S307294

Emergency Physicians

9

Gerald Fitzgerald

Catherine

It was 2 am in the morning. Catherine, in her second year of specialist Emergency Medicine training, unable to sleep, sat watching her children breathe. Their faces so familiar, yet confounded by the blood-stained images of the two children pulled barely alive from the tangled vehicle. It was the noise in the resuss room that most disturbed her. The crying of parents, the sharp rebuke of senior colleagues, and noises of the machines that seemed so out of kilter with frail humanity. She could hear that old professor. Keep your objectivity! Don't get emotionally involved! You have to be strong for the team. But what surprised her most happened that afternoon. In a rare break, she sat alone in the tearoom when the Director entered.

"Hi Catherine, I bought you your favorite coffee, sorry I couldn't add some whisky to it." She was surprised he even knew her name much less her favorite coffee. "You did a terrific job this morning. That was a tough gig. I hear those kids are going to make it, just wanted to make sure you do, too. Sorry to tell you those experiences stay with you, but they will make you a better doctor. I have used John Dryden's line to sustain me. 'I am sore wounded but not slain. I will lay me down and bleed awhile and then rise up to fight again.'"

They'll be OK, she thought. *Time to sleep.*

Introduction

Emergency Medicine (EM) was instated as a separate discipline several decades ago and its emergence reflected a substantial change in the way health systems across the world responded to acute illness and injury. 50 years ago, hospitals received acutely ill and injured patients by referral from their general practitioner or in the Casualty Department which was staffed by the most junior doctors. The paradox of the most inexperienced doctors attending to patients at their most vulnerable ultimately led to the development of emergency medical systems and the evolution of new

DOI: 10.4324/9781003292807-11

specialties including paramedics and emergency physicians (EPs). While this transformation is an undoubted benefit to the quality of patient care, it has come at a cost on both an organizational and personal level.

The introduction of EM as a specialty has made an impact. The growth in expertise and resources has undoubtedly improved the outcomes for patients suffering acute illness and injury, but by all measures it has come at a cost to those who have taken on this role. Indeed, this may have been predictable. As we sat around the table forming the Australasian College for Emergency Medicine (ACEM), we reflected on whether this new profession would have longevity as a career or was it a young person's game. Were those who sought to focus their careers on the acute phase of illness and injury a "special breed?" Would they relish the challenge and thrive, or would the nature of the work and exposure to life and death in its rawest form, ultimately lead to alternate career choices? For example, is Catherine's ability to pick up the pieces of her recent experience and move on to the next patient a reflection of her own inner strength that sets her apart from colleagues in other medical professions?

Emergency Departments (EDs) have become the front door of the hospital and the complex interplay of epidemiological, demographic, social, health system, and economic factors on demand, brought into sharp focus by COVID-19, have congested that front door, placing increased pressure on all of those charged with responsibility for acute care of the patients. At the same time, health systems have sought increased efficiency, reduced flexibility, and placed additional stress on key clinical decision-makers. EDs have become the "canary" for the health system, reflecting systems under pressure, and this has occurred in a broader context of social change in medicine including increased scrutiny and accountability. There is increasing pressure from growing demand, increased complexity of care, and increased community and professional expectations. Reductions in hospital capacity have resulted in access block. A point prevalence survey of EDs in Australia in 2018 (Australasian College for Emergency Medicine [ACEM], 2019) found that caring for patients waiting for inpatient beds represents more than a third of the emergency department workload. The introduction of performance indicators, such as the National Emergency Access Target, has contributed to the pressure placed on emergency physicians.

The growth in EDs has lessened the inherent comradery of small teams. Social change has also reduced the acceptability of coping strategies such as black humor, and the work intensity has reduced the impact of those rare quiet times when informal team building occurred, for example around meal breaks or after hours' social activities. Some thrive in this environment and grow from the challenges of building their resilience and finding techniques to manage these stresses (Manning-Jones et al, 2016; Yaakubov et al., 2020). Others find them confronting and require support, while others again suffer significant illness and psychological trauma (Chen et al., 2022; Somville et al., 2016. Unlike paramedics, the

ED staff do have some degree of control over their work environment, but they have little control over the nature of the work and the levels of demand or workflow.

In 1994, Lloyd et al. reported results from a survey of 395 emergency physicians across Canada and found 46% exhibited emotional exhaustion and 93% depersonalization. However, 61% were satisfied with their lives, and 75% were satisfied with their work. Increased age, quality of leadership, hours worked per week, and weeks worked per year were identified as negative contributors to mental ill-health. Similarly, Goldberg et al. (1996) surveyed 1272 emergency physicians attending the Australian College of Emergency Physicians (ACEP) conferences over the period 1992–1995 and found 60% exhibited symptoms in the moderate to high burnout ranges. However, they also identified a "survivor" group for whom burnout was a dynamic process capable of reversal; for whom coping skills can turn burnout around.

The issue of mental ill-health in emergency physicians is a worldwide problem. For example, Lu et al. (2015) surveyed both residents and attendees at two university-based emergency residency programs in the U.S. and found a burnout rate of 57% with no difference between residents and attendees. The burnout rate was associated with high rates of self-reported suboptimal care. DeLucia et al. (2019), in a survey of 526 emergency physicians in the U.S., identified a point prevalence of 15.8% with symptoms of PTSD. Jyothindran et al. (2021) found a burnout rate of 54% amongst EPs in the U.S. and the most protective features were provider appreciation and family support. Arora (2013) identified burnout rates of 60% amongst EPs compared to 38% for general physicians.

Truchot (2018) surveyed young emergency physicians across France and found 23% exhibited high levels of emotional exhaustion and 10% depersonalization. Similarly, Moukarzel et al. (2019) conducted a survey of 539 staff in EDs and identified a burnout prevalence of 34.6% among all staff but 50.7% among physicians. Kansoun et al. (2019) conducted a systematic literature review of burnout rates amongst all physicians in France and found higher rates of burnout, and in particular severe burnout, amongst EPs. Also in France, Estryn-Behar et al. (2011) surveyed a total of 3196 physicians, including 538 EPs, and found higher rates of intent to leave (21.4% compared with 17.4%) and burnout (51.5% compared with 42.4%) in the EPs. Work-family conflict and the quality of teamwork appeared to be the most influential factors.

Somville et al. (2016) surveyed EPs in Belgium and found one in three met sub-clinical levels of anxiety and 14.5% exhibited a clinical level of PTSD symptoms. They identified particular stressors including the death of young children, the frequency of severe and traumatic events, violence, and lack of social support, and suggested regular screening for symptoms and the creation of a supportive workplace culture as the most effective interventions. Chen et al. (2022) surveyed 15,243 EPs in China and found one-third suffered from depression. Adverse risk factors included being unmarried, a smoker, completing higher education, a long work tenure, poor sleep quality, and poor physical health. Liadova et al. (2017) explored burnout amongst emergency physicians in Moscow and found that all emergency doctors experienced symptoms of burnout at some stage, with 70% demonstrating risk-level symptomatology. They identified work-place stressors including night shifts, difficult patients, and job management as the principal stressors.

Darbyshire et al. (2021) explored the retention of doctors in emergency medicine through a systematic review of the literature. They found a range of factors associated with retention including teamwork, excessive workloads, errors, teaching and education, portfolio careers, physical and emotional strain, stress, burnout, debt, income, work-life balance, and antisocial working conditions. Several other systematic literature reviews have sought to collect and collate evidence relating to mental health impacts on EPs. Boutou et al. (2019) undertook a literature review on burnout among EPs and found rates varied from 25–77.8% dependent on the context, definition, tools used, and diagnostic cut-offs. They found EPs are at high risk from work-related factors including workloads, job satisfaction, and problematic co-workers, along with difficulty balancing personal and professional life. The rates were also found to be influenced by personality traits, coping methods, lifestyle parameters, and the presence of mental health disorders. Arora (2013) also identified work-related factors such as hours of work, years of work, professional development activities, and non-clinical duties influenced burnout rates, as did non-work-related factors such as age, lifestyle, and gender. Verougstraete et al. (2020) also conducted a literature review and identified burnout rates between 25.4–71.4% across 11 eligible studies. Non-patient-related factors such as large administrative tasks as well as human relationship issues were identified as predictors.

Attempting to uncover in-person factors, Pajonk et al. (2011) explored the personality traits of 274 emergency physicians and 245 paramedics. They found that personality characteristics are not homogeneous and do not differ substantially from other medical specializations. Additionally, they found that 50–70% were resilient and stable while 30–40% could be considered anxious and insecure. In a separate study of 487 German emergency physicians, Pajonk et al (2012) found low to moderate levels of stress-related disorders with 16.8% meeting the criteria for PTSD, 4.1% for burnout, and 3.1% for clinical depression. In this study personality type was identified as more impactful than the trauma the EPs experienced. On the other hand, there are personality traits that appear to be protective. Wong et al. (2018), in a small preliminary study, found that anxiety and working stress were strongly associated but individuals with high levels of grit were less likely to experience stress and anxiety.

These impacts have been brought into sharper focus by COVID-19. In the initial phases, EDs were the most visible source of assistance for a public dealing with the uncertainty of the environment. They rapidly became overwhelmed by the demands for care, testing, and reassurance while at the same time dealing with considerable staff absences associated with illness, caring responsibilities, or forced isolation following exposure. Those staff who remained struggled with the inability to provide comfort and support, rapidly changing protocols, and shortages of personal protection equipment (PPE) as important stressors (Hesselink et al., 2021).

Çalışkan et al. (2020) identified depression in 62% of 290 EPs evaluated in 2020 in Turkey. Rodriguez et al. (2021) found higher rates of workplace and home anxiety among academic EPs, citing the availability of PPE, rapid testing, and lack of clear communication. Claponea et al. (2022) undertook a systematic review of the literature exploring the impact of COVID-19 and found considerable evidence for additional burnout associated with COVID-19 across several countries and identified the lack of PPE and violence as issues related to organizational health. Kelker et al. (2021) conducted a prospective study across ten emergency departments during the initial surge of COVID-19. They found initial high rates of concern for personal safety and basic self-care and they also found high levels of resilience. Over the four weeks of the study symptoms of stress and anxiety improved but not burnout which remained at approximately 22%.

Given the complex work environment for EPs and the potential for particular people to seek out the profession, it is of interest to attempt to disentangle the likely complex interplay of external stressors and the personal circumstances and personality traits that influence the rates of psychological illness. Stehman et al. (2019) sought to provide a framework for understanding the factors known to influence adverse health, in particular burnout. They identified system-related causes including the demands of the electronic health record, long working hours, and substantial educational debt. Cultural issues such as the blame and isolation associated with errors, and clinical issues including the intensity of clinical practice and high rates of litigation, were also found to be influential. They also identified internal factors such as personality traits, the challenge of balancing life and work, and the presence of social networks and social support buffered negative impacts.

Bhardwaj (2022) describes the interaction of three domains in predicting negative impacts on mental health:

- Personal characteristics and traits including neuroticism, harsh self-criticism, idealism, and perfectionism in a social environment which includes work-life imbalance, overcommitment, and a lack of social support networks.
- Institutional influences including unprofessional leadership behaviors, racism and unconscious biases, microaggression, resource constraints, and lack of social support.
- Work-related influences including excessive workload and working hours, onerous documentation, fear of litigation, malignment with the needs of health administration, and loss of autonomy.

Distillation of these frameworks helps to provide the basis for understanding the range of factors that influence adverse health amongst emergency physicians which can form the basis of a comprehensive intervention program. Broadly, there are both external and internal (to the individual) factors. The external factors are those that derive from the nature of the work, the working environment, and the policy and organizational context in which Emergency Medicine operates.

- The nature of the work: Emergency Medicine occurs in an environment in which the individual provider is unable to control the workflow or the diversity and behavior of the patients. Providers lack the autonomy and control required to work as part of a team. Additionally, the overwhelming nature and insolvability of some acute health crises induce a further lack of control. Violent, drunk, and drug-affected patients pose a physical risk.
- The nature of the working environment: Emergency Medicine occurs through an intensive and continuous 24-hour environment necessitating shift work and long working hours. This pattern of work disrupts sleep patterns, meals, and relationships, removing known support mechanisms. On the other hand, support from colleagues and effective teamwork can help minimize the negative impacts as was the case for Catherine introduced at the beginning of this chapter.
- The nature of the organization: The culture of the organization and in particular its approach to the management of errors and the provision of personal support strongly influences the degree of psychological injury. Supportive cultures and support from colleagues have been shown to be protective.
- Public scrutiny and accountability: The degree of public scrutiny and accountability pressurizes the organization and the individual physician. It leads to defensive medicine and impacts management approaches and culture. The best supportive, no-blame, or just cultural endeavors can be readily undone by public and media targeting of individuals.

A variety of interventions have been trialed to mitigate the negative consequences of the work role and build resilience and the capacity for growth. For example, Chung et al. (2021) explored interventions in Emergency Medicine residency programs and found evidence only of small-scale success in reducing negative impacts which addressed limited factors. Schneider and colleagues (2019) explored the value of a specific intervention comprising multi-professional meetings and focusing on improved workflow. Results demonstrated partial improvement in work conditions and patient perceptions. McFarland et al. (2019) evaluated interventions aimed at improving mental health and found that a combination of strategies comprising individual-level interventions with system-level interventions that enhance workflow provided the most sustainable model for preventing and treating burnout. A systematic review of the literature explored strategies aimed at reducing the burden of the digital environment and its contribution to physician burnout. They identified 38 studies reporting interventions to decrease the digital burden and found improvements in burnout. Burnout reduction was aimed to be reduced by optimizing the technology, providing training, reducing documentation and task time, and expanding the care team (Thomas Craig et al., 2021).

Although the majority of research about EP mental health has focused on negative sequelae, some people thrive and grow as a result of the challenges they face. For example, there is evidence of posttraumatic growth. Yaakubov et al. (2020) demonstrated that posttraumatic growth was linked to posttraumatic stress for physicians in Israel, but not for nurses. They speculated that while physician growth was related to work experience, nurses' posttraumatic growth relied more on external factors. They suggested the impact may be gender specific. However, Hamama-Raz et al. (2020) found that while there was no difference between male and female nurses in rates of posttraumatic growth, women nurses exhibited higher rates than women physicians. They speculated on the lack of role models, reduced access to leadership roles, and the effect of dual family career responsibilities.

Emergency physicians have reported feeling a sense of achievement from the complexity of their role and satisfaction at navigating a complex and dynamic work environment. Crowe and colleagues (2017) suggest maximizing the potential for resilience and growth in this occupation includes giving EPs trust and autonomy to provide excellence in critical clinical care and the chance to provide mentorship and leadership. Manning-Jones and colleagues (2016) explored the factors that influence the rate of growth in a variety of health workers including doctors and found that humor, self-care, and peer support as well as supervisory support positively predicted posttraumatic growth. They speculated that the variations in social expectations of these factors influenced the various rate of posttraumatic growth observed in different professions.

Pathway for the Future

There is value in adopting a clear conceptual framework to help provide clinicians and system managers design, implement, and validate system-wide interventions. Some of the principal causes of stress derive from failures at macro-community levels including primary prevention, public policy, and health system design and resourcing. These are difficult to manage from within the ED although the ED is where the consequences are often felt. However, EPs can advocate for broader solutions. The broader social factors influencing demand are more difficult to modify.

Unless access block can be addressed, there is little prospect for a calmer and more stable workplace.

There are work-related issues characterized by the very nature of work, the work environment, and the organizational environments. Some are not possible to change. Emergency Medicine is always going to be the location at which people seek care during some of the most challenging moments of their lives. Traumatic events such as the death of children will always be associated with considerable emotions not only amongst loved ones but also amongst the providers, as could also be seen in the vignette. Others are partially manageable. Drug or alcohol-fueled violence may be difficult to prevent but policy and operational intervention may mitigate the risks to care providers. However, the evidence suggests that while the nature of the work can have an impact, most impact is felt by the challenges posed by the work and the organizational context within which the work is done. Multimodal approaches will be necessary to promote EP health, involving coordinated initiatives at the individual- and organizational-levels.

Some of the causes of distress would benefit from technological solutions to the problems. Many modern studies have identified the impact of electronic health records and associated regulatory and compliance requirements as having an adverse impact on the work environment. Research and evaluation are needed to develop and test more user-friendly solutions and to evaluate the benefit of compliance requirements. It is possible to improve the culture and operations of the workplace by, for example, reducing unnecessary duplication and creating a genuinely supportive culture, including peer support and leadership. Dealing with external scrutiny is more challenging. Service providers and their leaders need to develop techniques to protect staff from unnecessary or unwanted aggression including from those who legitimately or otherwise feel aggrieved.

Modern health service workplaces need to model the service values they exude towards patients, by applying them to their own people. To foster psychological well-being, supporting their people will require a multimodal and comprehensive approach that reflects the evidence where it exists but, just as importantly, is internally consistent. The core elements of any such program should include strategies aimed at the individual- and organizational-levels. At the individual-level, it should encourage self-awareness and self-compassion and support this through supportive structures, effective teamwork, and early recognition and support from peers. Catherine's supervisor showed compassion and support and even though the gesture may have appeared somewhat small, it made a big difference to Catherine who could then pick up and continue her work. At the organizational level, a culture of justice, tolerance, and support is needed, based on a philosophy of trust and reinforced by leadership, policies, and procedures. Such changes will likely not only reduce the negative impacts of the work-role and the context but enhance the potential for resilience and posttraumatic growth.

References

Arora, M., Asha, S., Chinnappa, J., & Diwan, A. D. (2013). Burnout in emergency medicine physicians. *Emergency Medicine Australasia, 25,* 491–495. doi:10.1111/1742-6723.12135

Australasian College for Emergency Medicine (2018). *Access Block Point Prevalence Survey Summary June 2018.* ACEM accessible on 6th June 2022 at: https://acem.org.au/getmedia/fa6f17ec-3926-4078-ac5c-529e7939e115/Access-Block-2018-1

Bhardwaj, A. (2022). COVID-19 pandemic and physician burnout: ramifications for healthcare workforce in the United States. *Journal of Healthcare Leadership, 14,* 91–97. doi:10.2147/JHL.S360163

Boutou, A., Pitsiou, G., Sourla, E., & Kioumis, I. (2019). Burnout syndrome among emergency medicine physicians: an update on its prevalence and risk factors. *European Review for Medical and Pharmacological Sciences, 23,* 9058–9065. doi:10.26355/eurrev_201910_19308

Çalışkan, F., Mıdık, Ö., Baykan, Z., Şenol, Y., Tanrıverdi, E., Tengiz, F., & Gayef, A. (2020). The knowledge level and perceptions toward COVID-19 among Turkish final year medical students, *Postgraduate Medicine, 132,* 764–772. doi:10.1080/00325481.2020.1795486

Chen, Y., Shen, X., Feng, J., Lei, Z., Zhang, W., Song, X., & Lv, C. (2022). Prevalence and predictors of depression among emergency physicians: a national cross-sectional study. *BMC Psychiatry, 22,* 1–8. doi:10.1186/s12888-022-03687-8

Chung, A., Mott, S., Rebillot, K., Li-Sauerwine, S., Shah, S., Coates, W. C., & Yarris, L. M. (2021). Wellness interventions in emergency medicine residency programs: review of the literature since 2017. *Western Journal of Emergency Medicine, 22,* 7. doi:10.5811/westjem.2020.11.48884

Claponea, R. M., Pop, L. M., Iorga, M., & Iurcov, R. (2022, May). Symptoms of Burnout Syndrome among Physicians during the Outbreak of COVID-19 Pandemic—A Systematic Literature Review. *Healthcare, 10,* 979. doi:10.3390/healthcare10060979

Crowe, L., Young, J., & Turner, J. (2017). The key to resilient individuals is to build resilient and adaptive systems. *Emergency Medicine Journal, 34,* 428–429. doi:10.1136/emermed-2017-206632

Darbyshire, D., Brewster, L., Isba, R., Body, R., Basit, U., & Goodwin, D. (2021). Retention of doctors in emergency medicine: a scoping review of the academic literature. *Emergency Medicine Journal, 38,* 663–672. doi:10.1136/emermed-2020-210450

DeLucia, J. A., Bitter, C., Fitzgerald, J., Greenberg, M., Dalwari, P., & Buchanan, P. (2019). Prevalence of post-traumatic stress disorder in emergency physicians in the United States. *Western Journal of Emergency Medicine, 20,* 740. doi:10.5811/westjem.2019.7.42671

Estryn-Behar, M., Doppia, M. A., Guetarni, K., Fry, C., Machet, G., Pelloux, P., Aune, I., Muster, D., Lassauniere, J-M., & Prudhomme, C. (2011). Emergency physicians accumulate more stress factors than other physicians–results from the French SESMAT study. *Emergency Medicine Journal*, *28*, 397–410. doi:10.1136/emj.2009.082594

Goldberg, R., Boss, R. W., Chan, L., Goldberg, J., Mallon, W. K., Moradzadeh, D., Goodman, E. A., & & McConkie, M. L. (1996). Burnout and its correlates in emergency physicians: four years' experience with a wellness booth. *Academic Emergency Medicine*, *3*, 1156–1164. doi:10.1111/j.1553-2712.1996.tb03379.x

Hamama-Raz, Y., Ben-Ezra, M., Bibi, H., Swarka, M., Gelernter, R., & Abu-Kishk, I. (2020). The interaction effect between gender and profession in posttraumatic growth among hospital personnel. *Primary Health Care Research & Development*, *21*, e35. doi:10.1017/S1463423620000377

Hesselink, G., Straten, L., Gallée, L., Brants, A., Holkenborg, J., Barten, D. G., & Schoon, Y. (2021). Holding the frontline: a cross-sectional survey of emergency department staff well-being and psychological distress in the course of the COVID-19 outbreak. *BMC Health Services Research*, *21*, 1–10. doi:10.1186/s12913-021-06555-5

Jyothindran, R., d'Etienne, J. P., Marcum, K., Ho, A. F., Robinson, R. D., Tijerina, A., Graca, C., Knowles, H. C., Zenarosa, N. R., & Wang, H. (2021). Association between burnout and wellness culture among emergency medicine providers. *Clinical and Experimental Emergency Medicine*, *8*, 55–64. doi:10.15441/ceem.20.074

Kansoun, Z., Boyer, L., Hodgkinson, M., Villes, V., Lançon, C., & Fond, G. (2019). Burnout in French physicians: A systematic review and meta-analysis. *Journal of Affective Disorders*, *246*, 132–147. doi:10.1016/j.jad.2018.12.056

Kelker, H., Yoder, K., Musey, P., Harris, M., Johnson, O., Sarmiento, E., Vyas, P., Henderson, B., Adams, Z., & Welch, J. (2021). Prospective study of emergency medicine provider wellness across ten academic and community hospitals during the initial surge of the COVID-19 pandemic. *BMC Emergency Medicine*, *21*, 1–12. doi:10.1186/s12873-021-00425-3

Lloyd, S., Streiner, D., & Shannon, S. (1994). Burnout, depression, life and job satisfaction among Canadian emergency physicians. *The Journal of Emergency Medicine*, *12*(4), 559–565. doi:10.1016/0736-4679(94)90360-3

Lu, D. W., Dresden, S., McCloskey, C., Branzetti, J., & Gisondi, M. A. (2015). Impact of burnout on self-reported patient care among emergency physicians. *Western Journal of Emergency Medicine*, *16*, 996. doi:10.5811/westjem.2015.9.27945

Manning-Jones, S., de Terte, I., & Stephens, C. (2016). Secondary traumatic stress, vicarious posttraumatic growth, and coping among health professionals; A comparison study. *New Zealand Journal of Psychology*, *45*, 20–29

McFarland, D. C., Hlubocky, F., & Riba, M. (2019). Update on addressing mental health and burnout in physicians: what is the role for psychiatry? *Current Psychiatry Reports*, *21*, 1–8. doi:10.1007/s11920-019-1100-6

Moukarzel, A., Michelet, P., Durand, A. C., Sebbane, M., Bourgeois, S., Markarian, T., Bompard, C., & Gentile, S. (2019). Burnout syndrome among emergency department staff: prevalence and associated factors. *BioMed Research International.* doi:10.1155/2019/6462472

Pajonk, F. G., Andresen, B., Schneider-Axmann, T., Teichmann, A., Gärtner, U., Lubda, J., Moecke, H., & von Knobelsdorff, G. (2011). Personality traits of emergency physicians and paramedics. *Emergency Medicine Journal, 28,* 141–146. doi:10.1136/emj.2009.083311

Pajonk, F. G., Cransac, P., Müller, V., Teichmann, A., & Meyer, W. (2012). Trauma and stress-related disorders in German emergency physicians: the predictive role of personality factors. *International Journal of Emergency Mental Health, 14,* 257–268. PMID: 23980490

Rodriguez, R., Montoy, J., Hoth, K. F., Talan, D. A., Harland, K. K., Eyck, P., Mower, W., Krishnadasan, A., Santibanez, S., & Mohr, N. (2021). Symptoms of Anxiety, Burnout, and PTSD and the Mitigation Effect of Serologic Testing in Emergency Department Personnel During the COVID-19 Pandemic. *Annals of Emergency Medicine, 78,* 35–43. doi:10.1016/j.annemergmed.2021.01.028

Schneider, A., Wehler, M., & Weigl, M. (2019). Effects of work conditions on provider mental well-being and quality of care: a mixed-methods intervention study in the emergency department. *BMC Emergency Medicine, 19,* 1–12. doi:10.1186/s12873-018-0218-x

Somville, F. J., De Gucht, V., & Maes, S. (2016). The impact of occupational hazards and traumatic events among Belgian emergency physicians. *Scandinavian Journal of Trauma, Resuscitation and Emergency Medicine, 24,* 1–10. doi:10.1186/s13049-016-0249-9

Stehman, C. R., Testo, Z., Gershaw, R. S., & Kellogg, A. R. (2019). Burnout, drop out, suicide: physician loss in emergency medicine, part I. *Western Journal of Emergency Medicine, 20,* 840–841 doi:10.5811/westjem.2019.4.40970

Thomas Craig, K. J., Willis, V. C., Gruen, D., Rhee, K., & Jackson, G. P. (2021). The burden of the digital environment: a systematic review on organization-directed workplace interventions to mitigate physician burnout. *Journal of the American Medical Informatics Association, 28,* 985–997. doi:10.1093/jamia/ocaa301

Truchot, J., Chauvin, A., Hutin, A., Leredu, T., Plaisance, P., & Yordanov, Y. (2018). Burnout and satisfaction among young emergency physicians. *European Journal of Emergency Medicine, 25,* 445–446. doi:10.1097/MEJ.0000000000000526

Verougstraete, D., & Hachimi Idrissi, S. (2020). The impact of burn-out on emergency physicians and emergency medicine residents: a systematic review. *Acta Clinica Belgica, 75,* 57–79. doi:10.1080/17843286.2019.1699690

Wong, M. L., Anderson, J., Knorr, T., Joseph, J. W., & Sanchez, L. D. (2018). Grit, anxiety, and stress in emergency physicians. *The American Journal of Emergency Medicine, 36,* 1036–1039. doi:10.1016/j.ajem.2018.02.021

Yaakubov, L., Hoffman, Y., & Rosenbloom, T. (2020). Secondary traumatic stress, vicarious posttraumatic growth and their association in emergency room physicians and nurses. *European Journal of Psychotraumatology, 11,* 1830462. doi:10.1080/20008198.2020.1830462

Correctional Officers

10

Olivia Miller and Dagmar Bruenig

Ash

Ash has been working as a correctional officer (CO) in a high-security prison for about two years. They were motivated to work in corrections so that they could support and rehabilitate prison residents. For the most part, Ash enjoys the work and looks forward to each shift. Ash is also aware that the job has changed them in many ways, and they are not always sure that this is a good thing. One incident from a few months ago has kept Ash wondering what the long-term implications might be. The incident involved a medical emergency in which Ash found a prison resident bashing their head against the floor so forcefully that blood and brain matter covered the concrete. Ash responded to the emergency following the appropriate protocols and was able to get the prison resident support in time to save their life. Afterwards, the staff debriefed about the incident and offered each other support but Ash was left rattled.

While Ash was proud that they were able to help the prison resident, they have had difficulty not thinking about the incident. They worry about what they could have done differently and replay the incident in their mind. Ash decided that they wanted to speak to someone about it and reached out to colleagues as they could best understand what the incident had been like. Ash's colleagues were supportive and so Ash felt somewhat reassured. However, Ash noticed that they were still nervous at work and vigilant towards similar situations. They decided to seek out support from their supervisor and their loved ones who reassured them that this was a normal reaction and encouraged them to access professional support through the employee assistance program, which Ash did. The prison resident injured during the incident reached out to Ash to thank them for their help. Over time, and through talking about the incident with colleagues and a therapist, Ash has been able to start reframing the incident as one in which they supported the prison resident as best they could.

DOI: 10.4324/9781003292807-12

The Role and Work Environment

As displayed in Ash's story, correctional work can be complex, dangerous, and potentially traumatic; but also rewarding. As a CO, Ash is tasked with caring for prison residents who often have complex needs and behaviors. While international differences in correctional contexts exist (e.g., Heard, 2019), the core tasks of correctional officers remain fairly consistent. At its core, correctional work involves three key tasks: custodial tasks, rehabilitative tasks, and emotional labor (Crawley, 2004). Custodial tasks are those tasks associated with maintaining security, for example, locking and unlocking cells. Rehabilitative tasks are those that aim to rehabilitate prison residents, for example, encouraging prison residents to make positive behavioral changes. And emotional labor refers to the emotion work that officers engage prison residents in, for example, empathizing and listening. Like other high-risk occupations, working under these conditions can impact officer health in both positive and negative ways. The salutogenic model (Antonovsky, 1996) views health as a continuum, ranging from dis-ease to health-ease. However, research with correctional officers has mainly focused on the ill-health experienced by people working in corrections, including medical and mental ill-health (Miller et al., 2022a). Understanding both ends of the health continuum is necessary to fully understand the complex dynamics of mental health and promote wellbeing effectively in this cohort. The following will provide a brief outline of research to date and then discuss more recent research in which the focus is on CO health and wellbeing.

Research to Date

Most research into CO health has been pathogenic with a clear focus on symptoms of mental illness (see reviews and meta-analyses by Butler et al., 2019; Dowden & Tellier, 2004; Finney et al., 2013; Regehr et al., 2021). This research has shown that working in correctional contexts around the world (e.g., America, Canada, U.K., Europe, Asia) is associated with symptoms of psychopathology including stress, burnout, posttraumatic stress disorder (PTSD), anxiety, and depression. COs are at significantly higher risk of experiencing mental illnesses like depression and PTSD in comparison to both the general population and other high-risk groups like firefighters and municipal police (Carleton et al., 2018a, 2018b).

Coming back to Ash's experience, we can see that they were demonstrating symptoms that may be consistent with a mental illness. They were vigilant at work, afraid of re-experiencing a similar situation, and ruminated over the incident. While this symptom profile appears to be mild, such symptoms have the potential to develop in harmful ways that may impact Ash's ability to function at work and in everyday life. If this were the case, Ash may be at risk of developing PTSD.

The current literature lists a host of factors that may contribute to CO mental illness, such as role conflict, perceived workplace danger, and exposure to critical incidents (Carleton et al., 2019; Dowden & Tellier, 2004; Spinaris et al., 2012). For example, prison and probation staff have been shown to have significant short- and long-term associations between PTSD symptoms and experiences of violence at work (Andersen et al., 2019). Critical incident exposure can also have a cumulative effect, with the risk of psychopathology increasing as critical incident exposure increases (Carleton et al., 2019). However, there are protective factors that may reduce a CO's risk of experiencing mental illness. These include peer, supervisor, family and friend support, a sense of job satisfaction, and the use of adaptive coping strategies (e.g., Butler et al., 2019; Cassidy & Bruce, 2019; Dowden & Tellier, 2004).

We know that Ash experienced the critical incident as distressing – they ruminated over the incident, were hypervigilant to similar incidents, and felt rattled. The literature tells us that prison staff commonly report feeling traumatized by workplace critical incidents (Carleton et al., 2019), particularly self-harm and suicide attempts (Cassidy & Bruce, 2019). Such sentiments are repeated by correctional officers in the qualitative literature where critical incidents are described as "[something] that doesn't leave you" (Garrihy, 2021). This is reflected in Ash's feeling that the job had changed them and their uncertainty around whether this was "a good thing."

Ash's risk of developing PTSD may be heightened for a few reasons. First, they may be experiencing role conflict as they desired to help prison residents but were unable to prevent the self-harm in this case. They also now perceive the workplace as dangerous, requiring them to be hypervigilant. However, Ash showed behaviors that may be protective, such as reaching out for social support. Social support from colleagues can be particularly useful because they are likely to have been exposed to similar incidents and have the unique capacity to understand what that incident may have been like. The fact that Ash is open to seeking professional support through the employee assistance program is protective because a professional can help Ash to process their experience and utilize adaptive coping strategies.

Contemporary Research on CO Health

While working in correctional contexts has been associated with a greater risk of mental illness, this is certainly not the only potential outcome. Experiences of health and wellbeing are also possible and can (and often do) overlap with symptoms of distress. However, CO experiences of health and wellbeing are less understood because they are under-researched in comparison to CO experiences of mental illness (Miller et al., 2022a).

We recently conducted a mixed-method systematic review on CO subjective and psychological wellbeing (Miller et al., 2022a). Subjective wellbeing is a sense of happiness and satisfaction with life (Diener, 1984), while psychological wellbeing is about optimal functioning including a sense of self-acceptance, positive relationships, autonomy, environmental mastery, purpose in life, and personal growth (Ryff, 1989). We reviewed 20 quantitative and nine qualitative studies and found that CO experiences of wellbeing were possible across international correctional contexts including Turkish, Canadian, American, Chinese, Nigerian, Polish, English, and Australian prisons despite the different cultural and political settings of these international prison systems (Miller et al., 2022a). COs exhibited moderate levels of life satisfaction and positive affect, and our qualitative synthesis identified elements of psychological wellbeing including a sense of personal growth. We recognized that various factors promoted wellbeing in COs including social support and a sense of job satisfaction.

Other limited research that was not included in our review examined wellbeing in prison staff more broadly. For example, Rousseau et al. (2008) found that a sample of 249 Canadian prison staff showed moderate to high levels of subjective wellbeing. They also found that positive relationships with superiors and peers were associated with heightened wellbeing. After conducting further analyses on the Rousseau et al. dataset, Aubé et al. (2009) found that observation of counterproductive behaviors in colleagues like parasitism, interpersonal aggression, boastfulness, and misuse of resources was negatively associated with wellbeing. Together, this research suggests that the quality of the workplace social environment can impact wellbeing. However, it is important to acknowledge that this research considered prison staff more broadly rather than COs specifically. This may impact the generalizability of the results as people that work in different prison areas may have different workplace experiences.

Job satisfaction may also be considered a positive health outcome for COs. Literature reviews (Lambert et al., 2002) and meta-analyses (Butler et al., 2019) of CO job satisfaction have found that work environment variables, particularly supervisor and peer support, promoted job satisfaction while personal demographic characteristics like ethnicity and gender had limited impact. In Ash's case, we know that they experience a sense of job satisfaction and purpose in their role as a CO. They enjoy the work, look forward to their shifts, and see their work as meaningful.

Further (admittedly limited) research has examined other health-related outcomes in COs including resilience. There is no universal definition of resilience, however, resilience is commonly referred to as the ability to cope, adapt, and adjust to stressful circumstances (see Aburn et al., 2016; Windle, 2011 reviews). The literature has shown that American and Chinese COs report moderate to high levels of resilience and that resilience can be heightened by hope, optimism, and social and organizational support (Klinoff et al., 2018; Liu et al., 2013; Williams, 2018). Ash has already shown resilience – they continued working to support prison residents despite feeling a sense of danger that engendered hypervigilance. Moreover, they continued working after experiencing a distressing critical incident and sought out support when they recognized that the incident was impacting them. Ash's support-seeking behaviors may enable them to bolster their sense of hope and optimism, thereby increasing their chances of remaining resilient.

Far less research has examined posttraumatic growth (PTG) in the corrections context. Tatebe et al. (2020) measured PTG in American emergency responders including law enforcement officers, paramedics, firefighters, and COs. The entire sample showed PTG scores indicative of significant growth, with COs showing the highest level of growth. Further PTG was significantly negatively related to PTSD. Demographic variables like years of service, ethnicity, marital status, sex, and having children did not reach statistical significance in predicting PTG. While helpful in showing that COs can experience PTG, this study did not provide much information about what variables might support correctional officers to develop PTG.

Konyk and Ricciardelli (2022) examined PTG in Canadian correctional officer recruits using a qualitative approach and found that participants recognized growth in their sense of personal strength and their compassion for others. However, the participants were correctional officer recruits, meaning they had not yet worked in prison as a CO. This means that their experiences of PTG were based on prior experiences unrelated to the corrections context. Nonetheless, moderate-to-high PTG is common for people in high-risk occupations (Wu et al., 2019), further supporting the notion that PTG may be likely for COs like Ash.

The preliminary findings of a qualitative thematic analysis of 22 semi-structured interviews with Australian COs found that COs experienced personal growth (Miller et al., 2022b). Interestingly, some domains of personal growth aligned well with the PTG model. For example, participants described a heightened appreciation of life and freedom and a recognition of their own personal strength. Officers also reported growth in their ability to understand and relate to other people through their work with prison residents. Other key themes suggested that adaptive coping and positive relationships with colleagues and loved ones may support CO wellbeing and personal growth.

To support the development of growth in line with the model of PTG (Tedeschi et al., 2018) and the other revised literature, Ash could engage in effortful rumination, seek out support, and hopefully bestow the event with meaning. For Ash, seeking support from colleagues and through therapy may help them effortfully ruminate on the incident and bestow it with meaning. For example, Ash has already begun to reframe the incident from one of distress to one in which they were able to support a prison resident. Over time, Ash may be able to recognize areas in which they have grown as a result of navigating the incident. For example, Ash may have a heightened appreciation for their own life having seen how quickly life can be jeopardized. They may also come to have a heightened recognition of their own personal strength given that they were able to successfully deal with such a difficult circumstance.

Mental Health Interventions and Strategies to Support Wellbeing

Ash's story and the literature strongly suggest that intervention programs are key in providing opportunities for improved mental health and personal growth in COs. Many prisons provide intervention strategies for COs to try to alleviate the burden of potential trauma. However, a recent systematic review and meta-analysis revealed that programs designed to help COs have been plagued by methodological issues (e.g., lack of control group or potential contamination of control groups), and Evers and colleagues' meta-analysis revealed programs had no significant effect in reducing symptoms of stress or psychopathology (2020). Notably, many of the programs were designed towards symptom reduction after a potentially traumatic event rather than prevention of negative post-trauma outcomes, potentially leaving COs more vulnerable to critical incidents. Those studies that did investigate prevention through, for example, formalized peer-support, did find benefit for the participants, but again, methodological issues prevent clear interpretation of the results. Due to these methodological issues and mixed findings, the authors concluded that while a range of psycho-education and intervention programs were available to COs, there is no evidence that these are successful in counteracting negative post-trauma. There may be several factors at play as to why this is.

While formalized programs may be offered in different prison settings across different countries, the continuation of reports of mental ill-health in prison personnel warrants further investigation. A recent qualitative study investigating Canadian Correctional Services Officers' opinions towards such programs and resources revealed a mix of suggestions for successful improvements of their mental health (Johnston et al., 2022). The areas identified as needing attention were system-wide adjustments beyond the workplace context with regards to consistent and funded access to mental health professionals specialized in the needs unique to COs, strictly workplace-related issues such as changes to work schedules that allow for more stability and predictability to reduce work-life balance stressors, organizational-cultural aspects such as improvements to staff-manager relationships, and lastly changes within the physical as well as a "virtual" workspace that would allow retreat opportunities from the floor to "take a break" (Johnston et al., 2022). Clearly, the actual programs appear less important than the concern about appropriate access.

These core findings demonstrate the complexity of stressors for COs and the need to address the reported issues holistically, beyond critical incident care and prevention and intervention programs. The theme of mental health stigma in the workforce relates to the observation in the literature that staff culture in prison settings needs improvement to support more prosocial behaviors and less negative talk between colleagues. For example, it has been shown that a sense of macho-culture is prominent in many prison settings that prevents open communication about mental health issues or uptake of available support programs (Aubé et al., 2009; Rousseau et al., 2008). Findings for the beneficial influence of a strong support system between management and COs have been reported previously (e.g., Bell et al., 2019). Ash's story showcases how a positive relationship with supervisors (and peers) can promote further access to mental health support. Ash's positive relationship with their supervisor allowed for the experience to be normalized and opened a dialogue about the incident. This was a crucial step for Ash to continue looking for help.

The observation for a dedicated physical space is interesting as previous literature had reported COs to just need to "have a bit of downtime" (Walker et al., 2017). A recent study in the U.S. investigated the efficacy of a yoga program focused on mindfulness and physical fitness and was deemed successful by the participants as it offered both a mental break as well as an opportunity to exercise (Smith et al., 2022). The request for a virtual space to retreat could be seen as an opportunity to more surreptitiously obtain support for mental wellbeing. A recent narrative review evaluated online intervention programs for public safety personnel including COs (Moghimi et al., 2022). Of the studies evaluated, the majority were published very recently (2021). Electronic cognitive-behavioral therapy programs – while sparse and relatively new in the correctional services setting – showed some promising results. However, the need for more education around these programs was also noted and in-person support was still ranked higher than online interventions, showing the importance of personal support provided through a therapist over a mix of educational programs and asynchronous interventions. Echoing Evers et al. (2020), Moghimi et al. (2022) noted the lack of pro-active programs even though enough evidence suggests that COs would appreciate preventative, rather than purely reactive programs. In line with Johnston et al.'s (2022) findings, Moghimi et al. (2022) suggested that programs specifically geared towards the unique needs of COs will have a better chance of adherence and completion.

One way of improving relevance and adherence to programs can be through the involvement of the target cohort. This approach was taken by Namazi and colleagues (2021) where they involved correctional officers in the design and execution of a one-year mentorship program. A follow-up study found that the uptake of this approach to designing a training program was high, and the program was also able to reduce burnout and medical factors commonly observed in COs (Kotejoshyer et al., 2021).

The program covered the first year of employment for COs and provided a mix of peer mentoring and health monitoring. The interesting approach here is that by involving COs in the design of the program, they received agency over their wellbeing and were involved in crucial decisions about their physical and mental wellbeing. Similarly, participation in decision-making processes has been shown to increase CO job satisfaction and buffer symptoms of burnout (e.g., Lambert et al., 2017).

Studies on other frontline workers have shown that giving and receiving social support is key for wellbeing and growth (e.g., Jurisová, 2016; Kang et al., 2018). The involvement of COs in an American study by Namazi et al. (2021) leveraged this approach through mentoring and improving work-related relationships and dialogue. This was also obvious in Ash's story. Ash worked in a supportive prison environment where there they felt comfortable seeking support despite the potential stigma associated with mental health struggles. As Ash's peers and supervisors offered support and normalized the experience, they were able to move on and find additional help.

A study investigating how social support might moderate biological factors commonly associated with accelerated biological ageing after the experience of trauma found that receiving social support had significant moderating effects on biological processes (Mehta et al., 2021). This is an important finding in the context of overlap between reported mental and physical health issues present in prison workers. While shift work, poor nutrition, and lack of exercise tend to be mentioned as contributing to ill-health in prison officers, it is important to acknowledge that the experience of traumatic events is not just the experience of the mind but transcends to the whole of the body with many different tissues affected by trauma (McLeay et al., 2017). Hence, programs and organizational changes that focus on education and the availability of social support may be key in overcoming access issues and a decline of mental and physical health in COs.

Conclusion

Mental wellbeing among correctional officers is an under-researched area that needs urgent investigation. Few studies imply the possibility of mental wellbeing and growth of correctional officers despite trying circumstances, and systematic investigations focusing on mental health rather than the absence of mental illness are sparse. The unique work environment of the prison setting requires holistic approaches for the improvement of mental and physical health for COs. An approach to staff wellbeing support that goes beyond the establishment of mental health training programs is needed to meet the unique needs of COs and overcome access issues. Physical and virtual spaces that allow for rest breaks and retreats as well as cultural implications in the structure of the organization must be considered equally before any successful training programs can be introduced that can improve the mental well-being of COs and allow for growth in adverse circumstances.

References

Aburn, G., Gott, M., & Hoare, K. (2016). What is resilience? An integrative review of the empirical literature. *Journal of Advanced Nursing, 72*(5), 980–1000. doi:10.1111/jan.12888

Andersen, L., Hogh, A., Elklit, A., Andersen, J., & Biering, K. (2019). Work-related threats and violence and post-traumatic symptoms in four high-risk occupations: Short- and long-term symptoms. *International Archives of Occupational and Environmental Health, 92*(2), 195–208. doi:10.1007/s00420-018-1369-5

Antonovsky, A. (1996). The salutogenic model as a theory to guide health promotion. *Health Promotion International, 11*(1), 11–18. doi:1093/heapro/11.1.11

Aubé, C., Rousseau, V., Mama, C., & Morin, E. (2009). Counterproductive behaviors and psychological well-being: The moderating effect of task interdependence. *Journal of Business and Psychology, 24*(3), 351–361. doi:10.1007/s10869-009-9113-5

Bell, S., Hopkin, G., & Forrester, A. (2019). Exposure to traumatic events and the experience of burnout, compassion fatigue and compassion satisfaction among prison mental health staff: An exploratory survey. *Issues in Mental Health Nursing, 40*(4), 304–309. doi:10.1080/01612840.2018.1534911

Butler, H. D., Tasca, M., Zhang, Y., & Carpenter, C. (2019). A systematic and meta-analytic review of the literature on correctional officers: Identifying new avenues for research. *Journal of Criminal Justice, 60*, 84-92. doi:10.1016/j.jcrimjus.2018.12.002

Carleton, R. N., Afifi, T. O., Taillieu, T., Turner, S., Krakauer, R., Anderson, G. S., MacPhee, R. S., Ricciardelli, R., Cramm, H. A., Groll, D., & McCreary, D. R. (2019). Exposures to potentially traumatic events among public safety personnel in Canada. *Canadian Journal of Behavioural Science, 51*(1), 37–52. doi:10.1037/cbs0000115

Carleton, R. N., Afifi, T. O., Turner, S., Taillieu, T., Duranceau, S., Lebouthillier, D. M., Sareen, J., Ricciardelli, R., Macphee, R. S., Groll, D., Hozempa, K., Brunet, A., Weekes, J. R., Griffiths, C. T., Abrams, K. J., Jones, N. A., Beshai, S., Cramm, H. A., Dobson, K. S., & Hatcher, S. (2018a). Mental disorder symptoms among public safety personnel in Canada. *The Canadian Journal of Psychiatry, 63*(1), 54–64. doi:10.1177/0706743717723825

Carleton, R. N., Afifi, T. O., Turner, S., Taillieu, T., LeBouthillier, D. M., Duranceau, S., Sareen, J., Ricciardelli, R., MacPhee, R. S., Groll, D., Hozempa, K., Brunet, A., Weekes, J. R., Griffiths, C. T., Abrams, K.

J., Jones, N. A., Beshai, S., Cramm, H. A., Dobson, K. S., Hatcher, S., Keane, T. M., Stewart, S. H., & Asmundson, G. J. G. (2018b). Suicidal ideation, plans, and attempts among public safety personnel in Canada. *Canadian Psychology, 59*(3), 220–231. doi:10.1037/cap0000136

Cassidy, T., & Bruce, S. (2019). Dealing with death in custody: Psychosocial consequences for correctional staff. *Journal of Correctional Health Care, 25*(4), 304–312. doi:10.1177/1078345819879752

Crawley, E. (2004). *Doing prison work: The public and private lives of prison officers*. Willan Publishing

Denhof, M. D., & Spinaris, C. G. (2013). *Depression, PTSD, and comorbidity in United States corrections professionals: Prevalence and impact on health*. Desert Waters Correctional Outreach

Diener, E. (1984). Subjective well-being. *Psychological Bulletin, 95*(3), 542–575. doi:10.1037/0033-2909.95.3.542

Dowden, C., & Tellier, C. (2004). Predicting work-related stress in correctional officers: A meta-analysis. *Journal of Criminal Justice, 32*(1), 31–47. doi:10.1016/j.jcrimjus.2003.10.003

Evers, T. J., Ogloff, J. R. P., Trounson, J. S., & Pfeifer, J. E. (2020). Well-being interventions for correctional officers in a prison setting: A review and meta-analysis. *Criminal Justice and Behavior, 47*(1), 3–21. doi:10.1177/0093854819869975

Finney, C., Stergiopoulos, E., Hensel, J., Bonato, S., & Dewa, C. S. (2013). Organizational stressors associated with job stress and burnout in correctional officers: A systematic review. *BMC Public Health, 13*(1). doi:10.1186/1471-2458-13-82

Garrihy, J. (2021). 'That doesn't leave you': Psychological dirt and taint in prison officers' occupational cultures and identities. *British Journal of Criminology*. Advance online publication. doi:10.1093/bjc/azab074

Heard, C. (2019). *Towards a health-informed approach to penal reform? Evidence from ten countries*. Retrieved from https://prisonstudies.org/sites/defa ult/files/resources/downloads/icpr_prison_health_report.pdf

Johnston, M. S., Ricciardelli, R., & McKendy, L. (2022). Improving the Mental Health of Correctional Workers: Perspectives From the Field. *Criminal Justice and Behavior, 49*(7), 951-970. doi:10.1177/ 00938548221081468

Jurisová, E. (2016). Coping strategies and post-traumatic growth in paramedics: moderating effect of specific self-efficacy and positive/negative affectivity. *Studia Psychologica, 58*(4), 259-275. doi:10.21909/sp.2016.04.722

Kang, X., Fang, Y., Li, S., Liu, Y., Zhao, D., Feng, X., Wang, Y., & Li, P. (2018). The Benefits of Indirect Exposure to Trauma: The Relationships among Vicarious Posttraumatic Growth, Social Support, and Resilience in Ambulance Personnel in China. *Psychiatry Investigation, 15*(5), 452–459. doi:10.30773/pi.2017.11.08.1

Klinoff, V. A., Van Hasselt, V. B., Black, R. A., Masias, E. V., & Couwels, J. (2018). The assessment of resilience and burnout in correctional officers. *Criminal Justice and Behavior, 45*(8), 1213–1233. doi:10.1177/0093854818778719

Konyk, K., & Ricciardelli, R. (2022). Tough lessons: Pathways toward correctional officer resilience and growth. *Traumatology.* Advance online publication. doi:10.1037/trm0000408

Kotejoshyer, R., Gilmer, D. O., Namazi, S., Farr, D., Henning, R. A., & Cherniack, M. (2021). Impact of a total worker health® mentoring program in a correctional workforce. *International Journal of Environmental Research and Public Health, 18*(16). doi:10.3390/ijerph18168436

Lambert, E. G., Hogan, N. L., & Barton, S. M. (2002). Satisfied correctional staff: A review of the literature on the correlates of correctional staff job satisfaction. *Criminal Justice and Behavior, 29*(2), 115–143. doi:10.1177/0093854802029002001

Lambert, E. G., Qureshi, H., Klahm, C., Smith, B., & Frank, J. (2017). The Effects of Perceptions of Organizational Structure on Job Involvement, Job Satisfaction, and Organizational Commitment Among Indian Police Officers. *International Journal of Offender Therapy and Comparative Criminology, 61*(16), 1892–1911 doi:10.1177/0306624x16635782

Liu, L., Hu, S., Wang, L., Sui, G., & Ma, L. (2013). Positive resources for combating depressive symptoms among Chinese male correctional officers: Perceived organizational support and psychological capital. *BMC Psychiatry, 13*(89). doi:10.1186/1471-244X-13-89

McLeay, S. C., Harvey, W. M., Romaniuk, M. N., Crawford, D. H., Colquhoun, D. M., Young, R. M., Dwyer, M., Gibson, J. M., O'Sullivan, R. A., Cooksley, G., Strakosch, C. R., Thomson, R. M., Voisey, J., & Lawford, B. R. (2017). Physical comorbidities of post-traumatic stress disorder in Australian Vietnam War veterans. *Medical Journal of Australia, 206*(6), 251–257. doi:10.5694/mja16.00935

Mehta, D., Bruenig, D., Pierce, J., Sathyanarayanan, A., Stringfellow, R., Miller, O., Mullens, A. B., & Shakespeare-Finch, J. (2021). Recalibrating the epigenetic clock after exposure to trauma: The role of risk and protective psychosocial factors. *Journal of Psychiatric Research, 149*, 374–381. doi:10.1016/j.jpsychires.2021.11.026

Miller, O., Bruenig, D., & Shakespeare-Finch, J. (2022a). Wellbeing in frontline correctional officers: A mixed method systematic review. *Criminal Justice and Behavior, 49*, 1559–1579. doi:10.1177/00938548221098976

Miller, O., Bruenig, D., & Shakespeare-Finch, J. (2022b). *"The job changes you": A reflexive thematic analysis of correctional officer wellbeing.* [Manuscript in preparation]. School of Psychology and Counselling, Queensland University of Technology

Moghimi, E., Knyahnytska, Y., Omrani, M., Nikjoo, N., Stephenson, C., Layzell, G., Simpson, A., & Alavi, N. (2022). Benefits of Digital Mental Health Care Interventions for Correctional Workers and Other

Public Safety Personnel: A Narrative Review. *Frontiers in Psychiatry*, *13*. doi:10.3389/fpsyt.2022.921527

Namazi, S., Kotejoshyer, R., Farr, D., Henning, R. A., Tubbs, D. C., Dugan, A. G., El Ghaziri, M., & Cherniack, M. (2021). Development and implementation of a total worker health® mentoring program in a correctional workforce. *International Journal of Environmental Research and Public Health*, *18*(16). doi:10.3390/ijerph18168712

Regehr, C., Carey, M., Wagner, S., Alden, L. E., Buys, N., Corneil, W., Fyfe, T., Fraess-Phillips, A., Krutop, E., Matthews, L., Randall, C., White, M., & White, N. (2021). Prevalence of PTSD, depression and anxiety disorders in correctional officers: A systematic review. *Corrections: Policy, Practice and Research*, *6*(3), 229–241. doi:10.1080/23774657.2019.1641765

Rousseau, V., Aubé, C., Chiocchio, F., Boudrias, J.-S., & Morin, E. M. (2008). Social interactions at work and psychological health: The role of leader–member exchange and work group integration. *Journal of Applied Social Psychology*, *38*(7), 1755–1777. doi:10.1111/j.1559-1816.2008.00368.x

Ryff, C. D. (1989). Happiness is everything or is it? Explorations on the meaning of psychological well-being. *Journal of Personality and Social Psychology*, *57*, 1069–1081. doi:10.1037/0022-3514.57.6.1069

Smith, H. P., Ferdik, F., Turner, A. L., & Radcliffe, S. (2022). An evaluation of a yoga program designed for correctional administrators and officers. *Journal of Offender Rehabilitation*, *61*(1), 37–60. doi:10.1080/10509674.2021.2017385

Spinaris, C. G., Denhof, M. D., & Kellaway, J. A. (2012). *Posttraumatic Stress Disorder in United States Corrections Professionals: Prevalence and Impact on Health and Functioning*. Desert Waters Correctional Outreach

Tatebe, L. C., Rajaram Siva, N., Pekarek, S., Liesen, E., Wheeler, A., Reese, C., Schlanser, V., Kaminsky, M., Messer, T., Starr, F., Mis, J., Bokhari, F., & Dennis, A. (2020). Heroes in crisis: Trauma centers should be screening for and intervening on posttraumatic stress in our emergency responders [Conference Paper]. *Journal of Trauma and Acute Care Surgery*, *89*(1), 132–139. doi:10.1097/TA.0000000000002671

Tedeschi, R. G., Shakespeare-Finch, J., Taku, K., & Calhoun, L. G. (2018). *Posttraumatic growth: Theory, research and applications*. New York: Routledge, Taylor & Francis Group

Walker, T., Shaw, J., Hamilton, L., Turpin, C., Reid, C., & Abel, K. (2017). 'Coping with the job': prison staff responding to self-harm in three English female prisons: a qualitative study. *The Journal of Forensic Psychiatry & Psychology*, *28*(6), 811–824. doi:10.1080/14789949.2017.1331369

Williams, G. (2018). Resisting burnout: Correctional staff spirituality and resilience. *Revista de Fomento Social*, *73*(3–4), 617–647. doi:10.32418/rfs.2019.291-292.1520

Windle, G. (2011). What is resilience? A review and concept ana-lysis. *Reviews in Clinical Gerontology, 21*(2), 152–169. doi:10.1017/S0959259810000420

Wu, X., Kaminga, A. C., Dai, W., Deng, J., Wang, Z., Pan, X., & Liu, A. (2019). The prevalence of moderate-to-high posttraumatic growth: A systematic review and meta-analysis. *Journal of Affective Disorders, 243*, 408–415. doi:10.1016/j.jad.2018.09.023

Military Personnel

Kaye Adams and Megan Fry

11

Rick

Rick is a 38-year-old male who served in the Australian army for ten years, deployed in combat zones including Afghanistan. He was medically discharged from the army eight years ago for a range of physical and mental health conditions including posttraumatic stress disorder (PTSD), major depressive disorder (MDD), and substance abuse. As these injuries were related to his service, he is in receipt of a veteran compensation pension. Prior to his separation from the military, he had been admitted for a 12-week inpatient psychiatric stay for detox, stabilization with pharmacotherapy, and trauma-focused therapy. Rick continued therapy for a year following his discharge, at which time he was assessed as stable and therapy was terminated. Rick reported that he found this treatment helpful at the time, but now feels lost, stuck, and frustrated with his ongoing difficulties. He is currently working as a civilian in the community and has a family but stated that he struggles with relationships and has a "short fuse." His wife urged him to seek help after a tirade that left his ten-year-old son terrified. He expressed fear of losing his family, resulting in feelings of hopelessness and an increase in suicidal ideation.

Psychological Treatments for Military Personnel

Psychological impacts of military service have been well documented, particularly since World War II (Scheutz, 1945), with PTSD identified as a significant risk for combat veterans (van der Kolk, 2014). Despite this knowledge, mental health issues for veterans are increasing, with anxiety disorders and depression the most prevalent (van Hooff et al., 2018). Emerging data indicates that mental health concerns are prominent not only for those who deploy into operational areas but also for those who do not deploy (Inoue et al., 2021). As the prevalence of females in military service increases, research indicates female veterans may be at more risk

DOI: 10.4324/9781003292807-13

of developing psychological issues and suicide compared to male military personnel in the U.S. (Adams et al., 2021), the U.K. (Finnegan & Randles, 2022), and Australia (Australian Institute of Health and Welfare, 2020). Veteran crisis line data identifies females report more experiences than males of military sexual trauma (MST), interpersonal violence, abuse, suicide risks, and self-harm (Dichter et al., 2021; Ramchand et al., 2016). Relationships are being recognized more readily as an important and primary part of the veterans' support system (Sherman & Larsen, 2018). However, Ormeno et al. (2020) identified that military families have more mental health issues than the general population and postulate this may be directly related to the challenges of a service lifestyle. These findings elucidate there are significant risks pertaining to the military lifestyle that need to be explicated beyond the current knowledge of the psychological risks and impacts of combat-related PTSD.

Much research to date on military populations has focused on and identified trauma-focused cognitive behavioral therapies as first-line interventions (e.g., prolonged exposure, cognitive processing therapy [CPT], and eye movement desensitization and reprocessing [EMDR]) along with pharmacologic support as secondary treatment (Moore et al., 2021). However, the modest treatment responses indicate that more understanding of military and veteran mental health is needed (Forbes et al., 2019). Hence, contemporary research is starting to explicate the nuances that make up the complex psychological issues within military populations and their transition from service (Castro & Dursun, 2019).

Multiple significant mental health impacts and vulnerabilities have been found to relate to the transition from military service to civilian life, which include: loss of the military support system, difficulties with disability and compensation processes, negative impacts of involuntary and medical discharges, and perceptions of public support (Castro & Dursun, 2019). Transition programs currently offered by the military tend to focus on support with employment programs to transition military personnel into the civilian workforce (Helfin, 2017). However, mental health, identity, and adjustment issues are also pertinent factors during this transition (Helfin, 2017).

Rick's initial pathway of recovery and rehabilitation was well managed by a comprehensive medical team and focused on his PTSD, depression, and substance use. This holistic approach assisted with stabilizing Rick's mental health and preparing him for his transition from the military, which was effective at the time and resulted in him being gainfully employed after service. However longer-term, his ongoing difficulties with emotion regulation, low frustration tolerance, angry outbursts, interpersonal issues, substance abuse, and suicidality endured, leading to the question "what is missing?" As adjustment difficulty is a common occurrence in military populations at transition from the military, there has been a shift in the research towards an exploration of exit triggers, discharge-planning, and the impacts of military culture and identity on transition (Kleykamp et al., 2021).

Military Culture and Identity

Social Theories of Military Identity

A significant amount of recent research has begun to focus on military identity using a lens of social identity and fusion theories. Enlistment into the military is a socialization process, which is where the military identity forms (Barnett et al., 2022). The military provides a culture and an environment where fusion can develop due to the familial nature, bonding experiences, and reliance on each other (Hart & Lancaster, 2019). Through military cultural practices, meaning can be created and maintained (Truusa & Castro, 2019). To grasp the complexities of the military identity is to first understand the conditioning process from recruitment, which is where military identity is built and which some refer to as "The Warrior."

Building the Military Identity

Mobbs and Bonanno (2018) describe the process of joining the military as a stripping away of civilian identities to transform and create a Soldier, Sailor, Aviator, or Marine. This transformation is a conditioning social-ization process, where compliance is demanded through fear and punish-ment (Mobbs & Bonanno, 2018). The military identity is developed and embedded with standardized group military values (Barnett et al., 2022). The individual self moves to a collectivist mentality, where the values of honor, loyalty, commitment, integrity, respect, and duty are indoctrinated (Atuel & Castro, 2018). Military training generates continual adversity, to create a "Warrior," which is mediated by creating a sense of team and comradeship that forms strong attachments within the military community (Atuel & Castro, 2018). This is an important aspect of forming the beliefs and behaviors of the "Warrior," as the extent that one fuses with the mili-tary identity, the more strongly they will embrace the military culture and desired traits of pro-group beliefs and in-group helping behaviors (Hart & Lancaster, 2019), which Swann Jr et al. (2014) have found to be a crucial element for the group to be family-like and worth dying for.

It is important to note here that there are many positive benefits of this conditioning socialization process, including:

- It enables an individual to work as an effective team member and to perform their duty and obligations of service.
- The military offers a family through its organizational security and purpose, which can bolster self-esteem and competence (Sugar, 2004).

- Military service can potentially mediate some adverse childhood impacts (van der Kolk, 2014), and there is a high prevalence of childhood adversity in military populations (Duel, Godier-McBard, et al., 2019).
- Military training ensures that the "Warrior" can run into battle and kill (Grossman, 2009).

The requirement to kill in service is an important consideration in the military conditioning process. Military training has been developed throughout history to ensure the warrior is mission-focused, hypervigilant, and able to overcome innate responses to flee and protect their kind (Grossman, 2009). As a consequence of developments in training and the conditioning of a strong fight response, there were significantly higher kill-rates between World War II (15%) and the Vietnam War (90%; Grossman, 2009). These processes are highly adaptive and effective for service and required in combat, but they pose issues during transition.

Difficulties with Military Identity during Discharge

Social identity models have been used to explore the difficulties with identity adjustment upon discharge from military service and the impact of transition stress that occurs in this process (Flack & Kite, 2021). A social comparison of "in group" with military and "out group" of civilians, which occurs in military training, can shape discrimination (Barnett et al., 2022) and cause pedestalling, which can endure after leaving the military (Binks & Cambridge, 2017). Castro and Dursun (2019) explain how the military identity of collectivism, self-restraint, low tolerance for ambiguity, and strong masculinity can impact when veterans attempt to integrate back into an individualistic community after service.

Binks and Cambridge (2017) found that difficulties post-transition are linked to conflicts with personal and social identities, loss of military identity, and disconnection from society. A strong and enduring commitment to service and military identity can make it difficult to engage in appropriate planning for a new career, new identity, and socialization as a civilian (Kleykamp, et al., 2021). An Australian report (Crompvoets, 2012) identified perceptions from female veterans as having a lack of an authentic veteran identity, described as feelings of being devalued, rejected, isolated, and displaced. This lack of identity then becomes a barrier to accessing services (Crompvoets, 2012). Whilst the difficulties with post-military identity adjustment are well researched and documented, there are currently no military-provided programs to assist military personnel adjust to civilian-life or that focus on unlearning the military cultural competencies that are required for service (Casto & Dursen 2019).

Changing the Military Identity

Changing the military identity is difficult. As discussed above, military personnel can be fused with this identity if it has served them well and kept them safe. It has provided stability, security, meaning, purpose, a sense of competence, and a sense of self. In addition, it is suggested that military personnel have a missed developmental period (Mobbs & Bonanno, 2018). The typical age of enlistment is 17–25 years, a time when individuals are still typically forming their identity and finding their place in this world and here the military provides concrete answers to existential questions (Mobbs & Bonanno, 2018). This impacts one's development of autonomy, an individual sense of self, and a sense of competence in the non-military world. Without the military identity there is an absence of any other sense of self as the pre-military self was cut away at enlistment. Hence, a program or treatment regime to assist adjustment in culture and identity would need to address this.

Like most military clients, Rick was fused with his military identity. He easily and quickly adopted the military values and in the military environment he felt accepted, a sense of belonging, and a sense of competence. He found meaning and purpose being in the military and liked the way everyone worked together to achieve a desired outcome. However, this created conflict for him after service, as he struggled to connect and tolerate others, particularly when things were not done efficiently, to the highest standard, as part of a team, or "right." He found living in community stressful and confusing and he couldn't understand what was wrong. Rick benefited from a different approach.

A Proposed Model of Individual Growth after Service

Understanding the psychological impacts of military service with the development of the military identity, the separation from civilians and community, the splitting of the self, the conditioned response to fight and kill, and the missed developmental period; we can create an atmosphere for change. If we train someone to take the safety switch off their natural inclination to save lives, and train them to "fire" and kill, we need to know the psychological mechanisms to put the safety back on (Grossman, 2009). To do this, we propose a therapeutic model of correcting and recalibrating military beliefs and behaviors, with a focus on emotional development and the opportunity for the military person to (1) develop their own sense of self and (2) explore and answer their own existential questions by learning about themselves, others, and the world in a new and different way.

To do this, we need to develop a concept of the pre-military self, the military self, and the now-developing self. This differentiation allows a process of integration to occur over time, which is important for long-term connection and well-being. It facilitates the opportunity to address any pre-military childhood trauma. It allows some distancing and separation from the military self, which is rigid and has fixed ways of operating. Finally, it allows for a new self to develop with an individual sense of self, autonomy, and competence to function in the world now. This process is also enhanced by separating the Military World from the Now World so that we can separate military beliefs and behaviors in an environmental context.

Through understanding and validating how and why the military identity develops, the pros and cons of this identity, and the protective mechanisms of this identity (for the self against punishment and for the group against danger), we can create the leverage needed to challenge unhelpful, ingrained military beliefs and behaviors. When we did this with Rick, he was slowly able to become aware of and understand the development of his military identity and the function of it. He could see the way he was fused to his military identity and how it was negatively impacting his life now. Techniques like chair work (a Gestalt Therapy technique, commonly used in Schema Therapy) were used to help Rick develop an awareness of the parts of himself and the coping mechanisms he was relying on to function day to day. His military self was redefined as a state of coping, rather than a trait or identity he could not function without.

By doing this, we have found that like Rick, our military clients are more able to connect to the more vulnerable parts of themselves, allowing understanding and processing of emotions; trauma processing of military and childhood experiences; development of compassion and empathy (to self and others); improved communication and interpersonal skills; and a widening of their window of tolerance. This process fosters a willingness to explore the world and become a "recruit at life," which allows the individual to start to develop a sense of self in the Now World.

Important Considerations for Individual Growth after Service

Arousal Levels and Limits

In our clinical experience, military personnel are chronically hyper-aroused, and their window of tolerance is narrow. They have been stretched by the military and they have learned to cope with and tolerate excessive stress and pressure, which is adaptive for service and protective in combat. The ability to push beyond all limits, detach from physical pain and all emotion and persevere under the most arduous experiences, is part of the military identity and it provides a sense of competence and acceptance. Hence, military personnel find comfort and safety in being switched on, hyper-aroused, and hyper-vigilant, and so when attempts are made to lower their arousal levels it can feel unsafe.

Our view is consistent with Stanley's (2019) reports about neuroplasticity and the impact of repeated experiences on the brain. The default wiring of a conditioned fight response in military personnel can result in "highly sensitized superhighways that get easily triggered" (Stanley, 2019, p. 93). As military personnel often do not complete a full recovery after a stressful experience (due to the nature of the military environment and culture), they remain in an activated state, enduring chronic stress activation, posing issues with sleep, relaxation, enjoyment, and connection. This can be why military personnel, like Rick, can be highly reactive, have sudden outbursts, use alcohol to self-soothe, and thrill-seek for the adrenaline rush.

To correct this maladaptive programming, one needs to develop new neural pathways consciously and intentionally (Stanley, 2019). This can be achieved by developing awareness and interoception of our somatic and emotional experiences; learning and understanding how to regulate arousal levels to widen our window of tolerance, developing an allied relationship between one's rational / thinking brain and emotional / survival brain, and developing self-control and self-regulation (Stanley, 2019; van der Kolk, 2014). To achieve this, we believe it is crucial to educate clients about why they are hyper-aroused, hypervigilant, detached, and disconnected from their bodies and that this information comes from understanding the conditioning effects of military service, not just as a symptom of PTSD. It is also imperative to assist military personnel to learn to recognize and accept their limits and break unhealthy patterns of striving for perfection and achievement, obsessing over tasks, analyzing mistakes, and tolerating abnormal levels of pain and discomfort. This price for ignoring messages from the body prohibits the detection of not only what is harmful to the self, but also what is safe and nourishing to the self (van der Kolk, 2014). Hence without this, military personnel can feel despair and frustration from never finding perfection, always being in pain, and never being able to achieve the unrelenting standards they are setting for themselves or wanting to see in others.

Anger

Whilst many believe there is a tendency for veterans to be angry, our clinical experience has demonstrated that veterans don't tend to _feel_ anger, but rather use the sensations of anger to armor themselves with posturing, ready to defend and attack as and when needed. This is again the impact of default and conditioned wiring in the brain (Stanley, 2019) and can result in military personnel acting out in angry ways (intimidating, bullying, attacking, scolding, belittling, or trying to control others) after service. This is often triggered by someone not following the assumed rules, failing to meet their internal standards, or perceiving disrespect they feel is owed. Again, by developing awareness, understanding, and reconnecting back to the feeling and sensations of anger in the body, we can assist military personnel to learn how to control the urge to act out in anger and instead develop emotion regulation and self-control skills.

Recognition

An interesting concept to consider for military personnel. Our clinical experience suggests that military personnel are instilled with the belief that if they succeed and achieve and meet the standards required of service, they will be recognized and valued by the community. This belief is first established at basic training and reinforced with graduation ceremonies and various military cultural practices in different countries, with holidays allocated to honor and recognize service personnel and their sacrifice. These practices and military training encourage a specialness in our service personnel, which perpetuates the pedestalling and separation from civilians. Hence, after service, military personnel can turn toward others to be recognized and may become triggered when this does not occur. Duel, Truusa, and Elands' (2019) study of public support in multiple nations identified that society can play a positive role in assisting veterans integrate into the community. However, if veterans do not trust or share with the public, they don't feel understood by them and so there is no bridge to facilitate integration or connection (Duel et al., 2019). It is therefore important that veterans learn how to step back down into the community and reconnect after service, whilst also recognizing their own achievements and reflect on their service with pride.

The Military Family

Military lifestyle is engrossing and demanding, which can create unique challenges for military families and potentially produce negative impacts on their lives (Ormeno et al., 2020). Families of military members are required to support the military, which can result in their lives revolving around relocations and the need to build self-reliance. Tensions relating to discharge (e.g., lack of routine and structure) and psychological therapy can also impact the family unit and hence it is important to consider the military family in therapy. If there is a lack of self-awareness and poor communication skills after discharge, there is the potential for tensions to be exacerbated as these difficulties are now tethered with close proximity to family (Madoc-Jones et al., 2018). In addition to coping with daily life, partners often become the carers of veterans with PTSD, resulting in them feeling invisible to the healthcare system; a system of people who do not fully understand partners' role and burden (Waddell et al., 2020). Therefore, providing counseling to promote healthy relationships and parenting support could potentially negate some of these difficulties (Ormeno et al., 2020).

The Way Forwards – New Programs and Research

Globally, there are many charity-run veteran organizations responding to the needs of veterans by conducting alternative interventions (e.g., equine therapy, adventure therapy, yoga, social support activities, etc.) using peer-run, veteran-specific programs to build skills and connections. Programs that reconnect veterans together can help them to feel understood, accepted, and regain a sense of belonging which can enable and protect the military identity (McDermott, 2021). As discussed in this chapter, this may only perpetuate a military identity that prohibits personal growth and community connection. Therefore, it is proposed that programs need to be more holistic in their approach to transition support.

Programs developed by psychologists specifically to promote post-traumatic growth in military personnel are beginning to lead the way, with positive change seen in longitudinal research programs such as the Boulder Crest Institute's Warrior PATHH. This program offers peer-run, non-clinical, long-term support using a growth model to facilitate personal reflections, self-disclosure, and connection with others. They teach life skills to increase community integration and promote emotional, relational, and spiritual health. Also, Stanley (2019) utilizes her own lived experiences and knowledge of military service to assist us in understanding the biological and neurological factors that underpin "The Warrior." From this research, a program – Mindfulness-based Mind Fitness Training (MMFT) – was developed that focuses on developing mind fitness to build interoception and widen the window of tolerance. This program has demonstrated improvements in mindfulness, body-awareness, and self-regulation practices for military personnel (Stanley, 2019; Haase et al., 2016) and may assist to help those currently serving in high-stress military roles (Jha et al., 2020).

Trials of novel group programs are being conducted, including a schema-focused approach that addresses the military parts of the self in conjunction with a growth model for adjustment and positive integration of the self into the civilian world (Fry, 2021). Groups can enable positive connections with other veterans and their shared experiences whilst facilitating a clear growth model for moving forwards and developing the post-military chapter of their lives. Transition support that addresses these prohibiting factors of the military identity with social connectedness and that also supports the broader family unit of the veteran is becoming recognized as an important aspect for a positive transition (Flack & Kite, 2021; Sherman & Larsen, 2018).

Many issues with transition between females and male veterans are similar, however, more recent research indicates MST, abuse, interpersonal violence, and self-harm differentiate as more significant factors pertaining to female veterans' mental health (Dichter et al., 2021; Ramchand et al., 2016). Veteran agencies specifically for women have just begun to develop and programs that provide support for women-specific issues should be considered. When in service, gender-specific challenges have been viewed as ill-managed or disregarded, posing particular issues for this group (Crompvoets, 2012). As cultural changes occur within society and the military, contemporary research will need to also consider and address any specific needs, including those of non-binary and LGBTQIA+ military members. As research emerges in these areas, prevention rather than cure can be possible in the future.

Conclusion

Whilst research into military mental health and well-being is expanding from traditional approaches focused on PTSD to more recent research investigating military identity and transition issues, this chapter brings to the forefront the role of the conditioning impacts of military service. By understanding the way that the military shapes an individual and the lived military experience of veterans, we can begin to explore what needs to be addressed after service and identify potential barriers to and avenues for facilitating growth. This chapter highlights some of the important clinical considerations when working with transitioned military personnel, in addition to their families and also female veterans. As the research continues to develop in this area, more preventative programs can be developed for veterans to assist them to shift and grow through these adjustment stages of life when returning from combat or completing service.

References

Adams, R. E., Hu, Y., Figley, C. R., Urosevich, T. G., Hoffman, S. N., (2021). Risk and protective factors associated with mental health among female military veterans: results from the veterans health study. *Biomedicalcentral Women's Health*, 21(55), 1–10. doi:10.1186/s12905-021-01181-z

Atuel, H. R., & Castro, C. A. (2018). Military cultural competence. *Clinical Social Work Journal*, 46, 75–82. doi:10.1007/s10615-018-0651-z

Australian Institute of Health and Welfare (AIHW) (2020) *National monitoring of serving and ex-serving Australian Defence Force personnel: 2020 update*. Cat. no. PHE 222, 9 October. Canberra, ACT, Australia: AIHW

Barnett, A., Savic M., Forbes, D., Best, D., Sandral, E., Bathish, R., Cheetham, A. & Lubman, D. (2022). Transitioning to civilian life: The importance of social group engagement and identity among Australian Defence Force veterans. *Australian and New Zealand Journal of Psychiatry*, 56, 1025–1033. doi:10.1177/00048674211046894

Binks, E., & Cambridge, S. (2017). The transition experiences of British military veterans, *Political Psychology, 39.* doi:10.1111/pops.12399

Castro, C. A., & Dursun, S. (Eds.). (2019). *Military veteran reintegration: Approach, management, and assessment of military veterans transitioning to civilian life.* London: Elsevier

Crompvoets, S., (2012). *The health and wellbeing of female Vietnam and contemporary veterans: Final report.* Defence Veterans Association. Australian National University, Canberra, Australia. https://www.afom.org.au/images/research/WOMENviet_fem_con_report.pdf

Dichter, M. E., Krishnamurti, L. S., Chhatre, S., Hoffmire, C. A., Monteith, L. L., Bellamy, S. L, Iverson, K. M., Montgomery A. E., Agha, A., & McCoy, I. (2021). Gender differences in veterans' use of the Veterans Crisis Line (VCL): Findings from VCL data. *General Hospital Psychiatry, 74,* 65–70. doi:10.1016/j.genhosppsych.2021.12.006

Duel, J., Godier-McBard, L., Maclean, & Fossey, M. (2019). Challenging missions: vulnerable veterans leaving the armed forces and promising avenues to support them. In C. A. Castro & Dursun, S. (Eds.) *Military Veteran Reintegration: Approach, management and assessment of military veterans transitioning to civilian life* (pp. 98–122). Academic Press. doi:10.1016/B978-0-12-815312-3.00006-1

Duel, J., Truusa, T., & Elands, M., (2019). Public support for veterans leaving the armed forces. In C. A. Castro & Dursun, S. (Eds.) *Military Veteran Reintegration: Approach, management and assessment of military veterans transitioning to civilian life* (pp. 216–240). Academic Press. doi:10.1016/B978-0-12-815312-3.00006-1

Finnegan, A., & Randles, R. (2022). Prevalence of common mental health disorders in military veterans: using primary healthcare data. *BMJ Military Health,* online first 18 January. doi:10.1136/bmjmilitary-2021-002045

Flack, M., & Kite, L. (2021). Transition from military to civilian: Identity, social connectedness, and veteran wellbeing. *Plos ONE, 16*(12). doi:10.1371/journal.pone.0261634

Forbes, D., Pedlar, D., Adler A. B., Bennett, C., Bryant, R., Busuttil, W., Cooper, J., Creamer, M. C., Fear, N. T., Greenberg, N., Heber, A., Hinton, M., Hopwood, M., Jetly, R., Lawrence-Wood, E., McFarlane, A., Metcalf, O, O'Donnell, M., Phelps, A., Richardson, J. D., Sadler, N., Schnurr, P. P., Sharp, M., Thompson, J. M., Ursano, R. J., van Hoof, M., Wade, D., & Wessley, S. (2019). Treatment of military-related post-traumatic stress disorder: Challenges, innovations, and the way forward. *International Review of Psychiatry, 31,* 95–110. doi:10.1080/09540261.2019.1595545

Fry, M. (2021). The military mode: a schema-focused approach to the military-to-civilian transition. *InPsych, 43*(4). https://psychology.org.au/for-members/publications/inpsych/2021/november-issue-4/the-military-mode

Grossman, D. (2009). *On Killing: The psychological cost of learning to kill in war and society.* New York: Back Bay Books

Haase, L., Thom, N. T., Shukla, A., Davenport, P. W., Simmons, A. N., Stanley, E. A., Paulus, M. P., & Johnson, D. C. (2016). Mindfulness-based training attenuates insula response to an aversive interoceptive challenge. *Social Cognitive and Affective Neuroscience, 11*(1), 182–190. doi:10.1093/scan/nsu042

Hart, R., & Lancaster, S. L., (2019). Identity fusion in U.S. military members, *Armed Forces & Society, 45*, 45–58. doi:10.1177/009532X17737021

Helfin, C. M., Hodges, L. B & London, A. S (2017). TAPped out: A study of the department of defense's transition assistance program (TAP): Chapter 4. In Hicks, L., Weiss, E. L., & Coll, J. R. (Eds.) *The Civilian Lives of U. S. Veterans: Issues and Identities* (pp. 61–90). Denver, Colorado: Praeger

Inoue, C, Shawler E, Jordan, C. H., Jackson, C. A. (2021). *Veteran and Military Mental Health Issues.* https://europepmc.org/article/NBK/nbk572092

Jha, A. P., Zanesco, A. P., Denkova, E., Rooks, J. D., Morrison, A. B & Stanley, E. A. (2020). Comparing mindfulness and positivity trainings in high demand cohorts. *Cognitive Therapy and Research, 44*, 311–326. doi:10.1007/s10608-020-10076-6

Kleykamp, M., Montgomery, S., Pang, A., & Schrander, K. (2021). Military identity and planning for the transition out of the military. *Military Psychology, 33*, 372–391. doi:10.1080/08995605.2021.1962176

Madoc-Jones, I., Hughes, C., Gorden, C., Dubberley, S., Washington-Dyer, K., Ahmed, A., Lockwood, K., & Wilding, M. (2018). Rethinking preventing homelessness amongst prison leavers. *European Journal of Probation, 10*, 215–231. doi: 10.1177/2066220318822245

McDermott, J. (2021). 'It's like therapy but more fun' Armed forces and veterans' breakfast clubs: A study of the emergence as veterans' self-help communities. *Sociological Research Online, 26*, 433–450. doi:10.1177/1360780420905845

Mobbs, M. C., & Bonanno, G. A. (2018). Beyond war and PTSD: The crucial role of transition stress in the lives of military veterans. *Clinical Psychology Review, 59*, 137–144. doi:10.1016/j.cpr.2017.11.007

Moore, B. A., Pujol, L., Watman, S., & Shearer, D. (2021). Management of Post-traumatic Stress Disorder in Veterans and Military Service Members: A Review of Pharmacologic and Psychotherapeutic Interventions Since 2016. *Current Psychiatric Reports, 23.* doi:10.1007/s11920-020-01220-w

Ormeno, M. D., Roh., Y., Heller., M. Shields, El., Flores-Carrerra, A., Greve, M., Hagan, J., Kostrubala, A. & Onasanya, N. (2020). Special concerns in military families. *Current Psychiatry Reports, 22*, Article 82. doi:10.1007/s11920-020-01207-7

Ramchand, R., Ayer, L., Kotzias, V., Engel, C., Predmore, Z., Ebener, P., Kemp, J. E., Karras, E., & Haas, G. (2016). Suicide risk among women veterans in distress: Perspectives of responders on the veterans crisis line. *Womens Health Issues*, *26*, 667–673. doi:10.1016/j.whi.2016.07.005

Scheutz, A. (1945). The homecomer. *American Journal of Sociology*, *50*, 369–375. doi:10.1086/219654

Sherman, M. D., & Larsen, J. L. (2018). Family-focused interventions and resources for veterans and their families. *Psychological Services*, *15*, 146–153. doi:10.1037/ser0000174

Stanley, E. A. (2019). *Widen the window: Training your brain and body to thrive during stress and recover from trauma*. U.K.: Yellow Kite.

Sugar, M. (2004). Warrior identity problem. In Flaherty, L. (Ed.) *Adolescent Psychiatry, V.28. Annals of the America Society for Adolescent Psychiatry*, *28*, 279–293, Medical Database. Routledge.

Swann Jr, W. B., Buhrmester, M. D., Gomez, A., Jetten, J., Bastian, B., Vazquex, A., Ariyanto, A., Besta, T., Christ, O., Cui, L., Finchilescu, G., Gonzalex, R., Goto, N., Hornsey, M., Sharma, S., Susianto, H., & Zhang, A. (2014). What makes a group worth dying for? Identity fusion fosters perception of familial ties, promoting self-sacrifice. *Journal of Personality and Social Psychology*, *106*, 912–926. doi:10.1037/a0036089

Truusa, T., & Castro, C. A. (2019). Definition of a veteran: the military viewed as a culture. Military Veteran Reintegration. In C. A. Castro & Dursun, S. (Eds.) *Military Veteran Reintegration: Approach, management and assessment of military veterans transitioning to civilian life* (pp. 6–18). Academic Press. doi:10.1016/B978-0-12-915312-3.00002-4

van der Kolk, B. (2014). *The body keeps the score: Mind, brain and body in the transformation of trauma*. U.K.: Penguin Random House.

van Hooff, M., Forbes, D., Lawrence-Wood, E., Hodson, S., Sadler, N., Benassi, H., & McFarlane, A. (2018). *Mental Health Prevalence and Pathway to Care. Transition and wellbeing research Program: Mental health and wellbeing transition study*. Department of Defence (Australia), Department of Affairs (Australia). https://apo.org.au/node/139561

Waddell, E., Lawn, S., Roberts, L., Henderson, J., Venning, A., Redpath, P., & Godwin, T. S. (2020). "Their pain is our pain": The lived experience of intimate partners in veteran recovery from PTSD. *Journal of Military, Veteran and Family Health*, *6*, 40–49. doi:10.3138/jmvfh-2019-0037

Warrior PATHH (2019). *Final 18 months results. Warrior PATHH: Volume 4*, Boulder Crest Institute, Bluemont, VA. https://bouldercrest.org/app/uploads/2023/08/Small_Digital_Vol-4_18-Month-Study-Final-Report-1.pdf

Child Protection Workers

12

Emma Malone

Molly

Molly was a 24-year-old child safety officer who had been working in the role for one year. She spoke about the impacts of the work on her in terms of sleep, relationships, and feeling unsafe in her own body, and specifically discussed a case that had stayed with her both in her waking and sleep life. This particular case involved Molly having to remove three young children from the care of their parents due to concerns of exposure to domestic violence, drug use, neglect, and emotional abuse. While removing the children, the father threatened to kill Molly and her colleague, and the police had to intervene to ensure Molly and her colleague could safely leave the home with the three children.

"I have nightmares about this case… I'll wake up screaming. It's weird though, cause often I am one of the children in the nightmare, reliving their traumas." Molly recounted going into the home of the children and how there were needles and dog feces on the floor. She reported remembering the look on the mother's face when she told her that they would be taking her children into departmental care. "The mother collapsed to the ground and started crying uncontrollably in the fetal position… I didn't know what to do… nothing in my training had prepared me to know how to respond." Molly remembers feeling profoundly anxious and overwhelmed watching the mother collapse and then the father screaming at her, threatening to kill her if she didn't leave his house straight away. "I remember feeling so overwhelmed with anxiety but having to get the three children as quickly as we could into the car, all the while having this parent screaming at us, detailing how he was going to kill us." Molly reported that on returning to the office, she had a quick conversation with her team leader, but that she was not provided with the support and guidance she desperately needed. Instead, she left the discussion feeling like she was lacking in skills and wasn't tough enough to do this type of work.

DOI: 10.4324/9781003292807-14

Over the last year Molly had felt increasing anxiety and hypervigilance, and would feel sick going to work on a Monday morning, terrified that one of the children on her caseload had been harmed or worse, died. Molly said her body would be "wired" after a day at work and that she found it hard to sleep. "My sleep has been so profoundly impacted… I'll often lie in bed, willing sleep to come, but it takes hours. And when I do finally go to sleep, I often wake up screaming from a nightmare." Molly discussed how she struggled to hear and witness stories of child abuse and neglect, day after day, whilst also noting how passionate she was about her job and her capacity to help young people. Molly reported that whilst she had recently started yoga and had found it helpful in terms of calming her body and increasing her feelings of safety, she felt overwhelmed by the level of risk in her work, the high caseloads, and the lack of support.

The Role of Child Protection Practitioners

Child protection workers are paramount to keeping vulnerable children and young people safe from harm. Across many parts of the world, the role of child protection workers involves investigating and assessing cases of reported emotional, sexual, physical abuse and neglect of children and young people, and intervening to protect them from future harm. Practitioners working in this field are not only exposed to severe cases of child abuse and neglect on a daily basis, they also endure staff shortages, high workloads, limited supervision, and exposure to potentially dangerous and violent situations. Child protection workers are placed in an impossible position as their work is underscored by three contradictory premises – (1) to keep all children safe from abuse and neglect; (2) to preserve the integrity of the family; (3) the general public should not become aware of instances where premises (1) or (2) are violated. In practice, often premise (3) is prioritized as the other premises are impossible to guarantee. Evidence of this is that workers often experience media, legal, and political scrutiny around the expectation to keep all children safe from harm (Chenot, 2011). It is therefore not surprising that for many practitioners working in this field, there can be emotional, physical, relational, and psychological costs.

Internationally, the terminology used to describe child protection workers, and the level and type of training workers in this field have experienced, varies greatly. Terms used include child welfare workers (Canada, U.S.) and child protection social workers (South Africa). In this chapter, child protection workers refers to practitioners in this field. This chapter will provide an overview of research in the child protection field and then review research exploring ways to prioritize the wellbeing of staff working in this high risk occupation.

Impacts on the Individual

Studies on practitioners working in the child protection sector have identified high levels of burnout, secondary traumatic stress, and compassion fatigue. This body of literature has found common impacts on child protection practitioners include an increase in anxiety (Gibbs, 2001), hypervigilance, sleep disturbance (Jirek, 2015), dissociation, physical health problems (Kim & Kao, 2014), and relational difficulties (McFadden, 2020). Whilst there have been limitations in the research, namely selection bias, small sample sizes, and differing terminology for the impacts, the research in this area identifies that stress, burnout, and trauma responses are endemic in child protection work (Conrad & Kellar-Guenther, 2006; Hunt et al., 2016; Kim & Kao, 2014; Lamothe et al., 2018; Regehr et al., 2004).

The Center for Advanced Studies in Child Welfare (CASCW) and the Minnesota Association of County Social Service Administrators (MACSSA) conducted research with 862 front-line and supervising child protection practitioners exploring the wellbeing of staff and their beliefs around continuing in the workforce (2016). They found that 68% of the respondents felt overwhelmed by their work, with 83% reporting experiencing secondary traumatic stress. Over a fifth of the respondents reported that they were seeking employment elsewhere. These findings align with research by Conrad and Kellar-Gunther (2006) which found that 50% of the 363 child protection workers in their study reported high to very high levels of compassion fatigue.

A unique challenge in this field is that practitioners are not only at risk of developing secondary trauma but also, in the course of their work, experiencing direct trauma. For example, an Australian study interviewed 50 child protection workers about their exposure to intimidating and hostile behavior in their work (Stanley et al., 2002). The findings identified high levels of intimidation and violence towards workers, including threats to themselves and family members, threats of sexual assault, and threats including the use of knives. In addition, many workers reported being victims of direct assaults including hair pulling, shoving, and attempted strangulation (Stanley et al., 2002). This study noted that trauma responses were evident in workers, particularly those who experienced high levels of trauma with low supervisory support. Similar experiences were noted in a study of 590 social workers (72% child protection workers) looking at exposure to hostile parents (Hunt et al., 2016). High levels of exposure to violent behavior were reported, including intimidation, death threats, and physical violence, with the resulting impacts of increased sleep disturbances, stress, and anxiety.

As is evident in the case of Molly, there can often be bodily responses to child protection work. Embodied impacts of trauma work have gained increased attention over the last decade. For example, a longitudinal study of 406 social workers in the U.S. found that workers with higher levels of burnout experienced higher levels of physical health complaints, including sleep disturbances, gastrointestinal problems, headaches, and respiratory infections (Kim et al., 2011). In addition, practitioners who reported higher burnout levels experienced a larger decline in their overall physical health over a one-year period. Similarly, Jirek (2015) found embodied impacts including numbing, nausea, body aches, headaches, diarrhea, and tension throughout the body. Taken together, these studies demonstrate how child protection workers are regularly faced with both direct and vicarious experiences of trauma, impacting both their psychological and physical health.

System-wide Impacts

Whilst the cost on the individual worker's life can be profound, on a systemic level these impacts lead to high rates of sick days, performance problems, low job satisfaction, and turnover (Lamothe et al., 2018; Truter et al., 2018). In America, data on the turnover rates across states and jurisdictions over the last 15 years place the average annual turnover rate between 20–40%, with some states being as high as 65% (Munro, 2011; Auerbach et al., 2010). For the young people and families involved in the child protection systems, these worker and system-wide impacts can be devastating and, sometimes, deadly.

Given the need for relational stability and consistency in child development, research has found that child protection systems that are fractured and in crisis lead to profound harm in the lives of vulnerable people (Ellett et al., 2007; Strolin-Goltzman et al., 2010). For example, a study exploring the experiences of young people (n=25) in the foster care system in New York found common responses to worker turnover included feelings of physical and emotional instability, a loss of trust in others, and a disruption in the development of safe, healthy relationships (Strolin-Goltzman et al., 2010). In Australia alone, there have been more than 30 inquiries into the child protection system in the last 25 years, with most inquiries occurring following the death of a young person or an apparent failure in the system. The findings from these inquiries have identified high workloads, high turnover, and poor supervision playing a role in system failings (Goddard & Hunt, 2011).

Positive Change through Child Protection Work

While research has identified that trauma responses are endemic in child protection work, research has also identified the potential for positive outcomes, namely increased resilience, PTG, and vicarious post traumatic growth (VPTG) (e.g., see McFadden, 2020; Truter et al., 2018). Several studies have found that as levels of distress in child protection workers increase, so too do levels of PTG (Regehr et al., 2004). This research, whilst not identified to detract from how difficult and overwhelming it can be to work in this profession, provides hope for practitioners in the field as positive change is posited to occur. It is argued that growth may occur in child protection practitioners by actively engaging with and processing work-related trauma and deriving meaning. Studies on VPTG in other fields have found improvements in relationships (Barrington & Shakespeare-Finch, 2013), sense of self (Manning-Jones et al., 2016), and feelings of workplace competence (Manning-Jones et al., 2015). However, caution needs to be taken when analyzing the studies of both trauma and PTG as most research conducted on child protection workers is with practitioners currently in the profession. Levels of burnout and trauma responses may therefore be significantly underreported due to the high rates of turnover, and data may be skewed towards those who thrive in this stressful work environment. Collectively, this body of research identifies high rates of physical and psychological health impacts in this line of work, coupled with the possibility of increased resilience and PTG. Consequently, it is crucial to understand both the risk and protective factors in this work that can help protect child protection workers and promote resilience and growth.

Risk and Protective Factors

Given the often-devastating impacts of child protection work, and the flow-on effects for the young people these systems serve, research has explored the role of individual and systemic risk and protective factors in the work. Common factors found in the research include role overload, supervision, and exposure to distressing material (Kong, 2005; Mor Barak et al., 2009). A study of child protection staff ($n=156$) in Canada explored the relationships between post traumatic distress and growth in workers and individual and organizational factors (Regehr et al., 2004). They found that the strongest predictor of distress in child protection workers was organizational factors, including high workloads and challenging clients. These findings are comparable to a study of child protection workers ($n=268$) in South Korea that explored the relationships between risk and protective factors, burnout, intent to leave, and job satisfaction (Chung & Choo, 2019). A structural path analysis identified that emotional exhaustion, high workloads, safety concerns, and secondary traumatic stress all increased intent to leave.

Similarly, a meta-analysis exploring workers intentions to leave in the U.S. child protection sector identified that the strongest predictors were organizational support, stress, safety concerns, role conflict, job demand, emotional exhaustion and depersonalization, organizational commitment, and job satisfaction (Kim & Kao, 2014). Organizational support was also found to be crucial to experiences of both burnout and resilience in a phenomenological study in Northern Ireland with child protection workers (McFadden et al., 2018). The workers reported feeling more resilient and able to cope with the work pressures when they had supportive managers, including supportive, regular, and caring supervision. Limited support and supervision were identified to lead to high absenteeism and turnover. Similar to Molly's experience, for many child protection workers the supervision and support provided are insufficient.

Whilst overwhelmingly the research points towards the role of organizational factors, some individual factors have also been identified, including age, worker well-being, tenure, training, coping styles, and job satisfaction (e.g., see Kim & Kao, 2014; McFadden et al., 2015). Many of the studies on individual factors identified the role of coping mechanisms in protecting workers, particularly self-awareness and active engagement in coping strategies. This is important to note as, just like in the case of Molly, workers often have existing skills and strategies available to help them navigate the difficulties of child protection work; however, often they require the support and training of senior workers including supervisors. Interestingly, in trying to understand how workers cope in this field, resilience commonly arises; however, how the term is conceptualized and measured varies greatly. In addition, there is backlash in the profession to the concept of resilience as it is often defined as an inherent personality trait, ignoring the relational, time-specific, and context-specific drivers that can promote or hinder resilience within a person's life (Rutter, 1990). Whilst often viewed as an individual factor, research in the child welfare field has highlighted the relational aspects of resilience, namely that supportive relationships in the workplace can promote more resilience towards stress or, alternatively, lead to burnout (Kinman & Grant, 2011; McFadden, 2020; McFadden et al., 2015).

Taken together, the research on the impacts of child protection work and the risk and protective factors points to many important areas that need to be addressed to improve the experiences of workers in this system. For change to occur, intervention needs to be targeted at both the individual and organizational levels.

Individual-level Strategies

Given the embodied impacts of trauma, mental health strategies over the last decade have broadened to include a focus on body-based interventions in helping to reduce trauma symptoms and increase engagement in life. Yoga is one such body-based intervention that may be a promising coping mechanism for practitioners who are faced with highly stressful work. Yoga involves breath exercises, physical poses, and movement, and is argued to increase safety in the body and build capacity to regulate the overwhelming bodily and emotional states impacted by trauma (van der Kolk, 2014). Yoga has been found to be an effective treatment approach for a wide range of difficulties including stress, anxiety, depression, and

PTSD (Kelly et al., 2021; Macy et al., 2015; Pascoe & Bauer, 2015; Taylor et al., 2020). Some studies with child protection workers have noted the role of yoga in helping workers feel more relaxed and calm (e.g., see Truter et al., 2018). A systematic review exploring the use of yoga in stress reduction across professions and countries including Australia, Taiwan, Iraq, the U.S., and the U.K. found positive changes on measures of physical and psychological stress (Sharma, 2014). These changes included reductions in stress and anxiety, improved heart rate variability, and decreased mood disturbances. A more recent study with veteran women who had experienced military sexual trauma found improvements in self-compassion and shame, sleep, and capacity to regulate affect following engagement in trauma-informed yoga (Braun et al., 2021).

Given the limited research specific to this field, research into the use of yoga with survivors of direct trauma sheds light on the potential for yoga to help child protection workers. In particular, research into the use of trauma-sensitive yoga with people who have experienced single event and/or complex trauma has found positive changes through the use of yoga (Braun et al., 2021; Crews et al., 2016; Gladden et al., 2022; Ong et al., 2019). For example, a long-term follow-up study using yoga with women ($n=60$) who had experienced complex trauma and had treatment-resistant PTSD found that those who had continued regular yoga practice experienced decreased depressive symptoms and trauma symptomatology (Rhodes et al., 2016). Similar findings were identified in a randomized controlled trial using yoga with people ($n= 94$) who had survived a motor vehicle accident (Yi et al., 2022). For participants who engaged in the yoga intervention, there were significant changes in depression, anxiety, thought intrusion, and avoidance. A recent systematic review and meta-analysis found yoga to be an effective adjunctive treatment for people exposed to trauma, including people in trauma-exposed occupations (Taylor et al., 2020).

Whilst studies have often been limited by small sample sizes and a lack of standardized yoga interventions, the research on yoga suggests that it can be helpful in reducing anxiety, regulating emotional arousal, and creating safety in the body. It, therefore, holds promise as a form of self-care that child protection workers can use to cope with the many impacts of their work. As can be seen in the case of Molly, regular engagement in yoga helped to reduce some of the impacts of the work, including anxiety and hypervigilance, whilst allowing her to feel safe within her own body. However, studies have continued to highlight that individual practices alone are not enough to negate the impacts of child protection work.

Organizational-level Strategies

A continued sentiment echoed in the research has been that placing the responsibility of worker wellbeing solely on individual workers undermines the greater systemic issues that occur in child protection work. Whilst there is a part for each individual to play in looking after themselves in the profession, given the knowledge that this work has negative impacts on practitioners implies that this is a common and shared experience. There is a duty of care for organizations and child protection systems to address the known risks and difficulties on a systemic level. Supervision is one such area that has been found to play a role in the wellbeing of child protection workers and decrease turnover (e.g., McFadden et al., 2015).

As identified, child protection work can be highly distressing and emotive, both through exposure to details of child abuse and neglect, and through having to repeatedly engage with adults who may have difficult relational and response dynamics, including intimidation and threats to harm (Hunt et al., 2016). To cope, many practitioners may employ defensive coping mechanisms such as avoidance or dissociation which may, in the short term, provide some level of stress reduction, but have ongoing issues for their own wellbeing and for the provision of responsive casework (Stanley et al., 2002). Given the complexity of working in this field, supervision is crucial in supporting workers. Studies on supervision across many professions working with victims of trauma have found that supervision is a key component to mitigating the impacts of the work. Many studies have found a reduction in burnout levels when workers have experienced supportive supervision (e.g., see Itzhaky & Aviad-Hiebloom, 1998; McFadden, 2020; Mor Barak et al., 2009), with some studies finding that supportive supervision can lead to resilience and growth in practitioners (Ben-Porat et al., 2020; Brockhouse et al., 2011; McFadden, 2020) and an increase in work commitment (Barth et al., 2008). In addition, supervision that is scheduled on a regular basis has been found to lead to higher rates of retention and worker satisfaction (Lietz & Rounds, 2009).

This is an area that warrants further research specific to child protection as there are few high-quality studies conducted, and often the findings have been mixed (Carpenter et al., 2013). For example, some studies have found that supervision has not reduced levels of burnout and stress in social workers (e.g., see Um & Harrison, 1998; Regehr et al., 2004). A closer examination of studies exploring the role of supervision in child protection work suggests that it is the *type* of supervision that is key (e.g., see McFadden, 2020). Supervision that focuses on administrative tasks, worker performance, and accountability has not been found to reduce levels of worker distress. For example, a qualitative study with 22 child protection workers in rural Australia identified that for workers who reported little supervision or task-focused supervision, supervision led to feelings of anger and disappointment (Gibbs, 2001). Ferguson (2006) and Munro (2011) have both criticized the systems of supervision in child protection, arguing that in response to system failures, including child deaths, focus on procedural and reporting requirements have resulted in supervision that does not provide worker support or space for reflection. This type of supervision is evident in Molly's case, as the brief supervision she received following the family group meeting did not provide her with support or processing the experience, leaving her feeling worse and questioning her suitability for the work.

So, what then are the key components needed in supervision to help support child protection workers? A meta-analysis on supervision across different professions in the U.S. found that supervision that included social and emotional support, task guidance, and interpersonal interaction was linked to positive outcomes in workers (Mor Barak et al., 2009). Munro (2011) identified that supervision in child protection work needed to not only provide emotional support but also allow space for reflective practice. Kinman and Grant (2011) argued that supervision that encouraged reflexive and reflective practice increased resilience in the workplace. For this type of supervision to occur, the supervisory relationship needs to be safe and of a good quality. The relationship between the supervisor and the child protection worker has been found to be key in supporting workers and playing a role in fostering resilience or contributing towards burnout (McFadden, 2020). Exploring the experiences of child protection workers who chose to leave the work (n=15) and who chose to stay (n=15), the importance of the supervisory relationship was highlighted in helping keep workers in the field and protecting them from burnout (McFadden, 2020). Of particular note in the supervisory relationship were supervisors who demonstrated care and commitment, understood the inherent pressures of the work, and identified workers' strengths. This type of supportive supervision, which not only identifies workers' strengths but also identifies challenges in a reflective process, has been found to deepen practitioners' work and keep them in the child protection workforce (McFadden, 2020).

Furthermore, given the high levels of trauma experienced by clients and practitioners in the child welfare system, trauma-informed supervision is argued to be crucial in providing support to workers in this field. Surprisingly, given the abundance of research over the last ten years on trauma-informed care (TIC), particularly in child welfare systems across the U.S. (e.g., see Barto et al., 2018; Connell et al., 2019; Lang et al., 2016), there is very little research which has explored trauma-informed-supervision in child protection. Nevertheless, a recent paper on trauma-informed child protection supervision made several important recommendations (Collins-Camargo & Antle, 2018):

Ensuring a trauma focus in all child protection work, including understanding how trauma impacts on clients and how they need to be supported. In applying this to the case of Molly, this could involve her supervisor asking Molly how trauma may be playing a role in the responses of the parents to child safety's intervention, and whether any trauma assessments or trauma-specific interventions need to be actioned (e.g., referrals).

Reflective supervision that is aimed at helping supervisees process the complexity of their roles. In supervision for Molly, this could include questioning from her supervisor to enable Molly to reflect on her interactions with the parents, the effectiveness of her communication, and what it was like for

Molly to witness the responses of the parents. A key part of this is the supervisor responding empathically, providing containment of Molly's emotional responses, which will help enable Molly to start processing the work-related trauma.

Active engagement with clients, which includes a supervisor who will go into the field with staff. For Molly, this could involve her supervisor joining her on challenging home visits and meetings to help provide insight into family dynamics and also help to hold the trauma.

Facilitating practice that is evidence-informed, including the incorporation of new evidence and practice into work. Through team culture and regular team meetings, Molly's supervisor could introduce new evidenced, informed trauma research and practice to Molly and her colleagues.

Prevention and support for trauma workers, including acknowledging the risks of the work, embedding practices to minimize impacts, support and empathy to workers, and acknowledgement of strengths. Molly's supervisor may address this element by openly discussing secondary and vicarious trauma in team meetings (creating a team culture that normalizes experiences of secondary and vicarious trauma); scheduling self-care activities at the end of team meetings; and acknowledging the strengths of the team.

Trauma-informed training and support for supervisors. For Molly's supervisor it is crucial for them to have had training in trauma (including secondary and vicarious trauma) and have good support systems in place both within the organization and externally. In doing so, Molly's supervisor can normalize and empathize with the impacts of the work, include discussions of this and self-care in supervision, and manage workloads based on the risk of trauma responses and burnout in workers.

Ultimately, regular supervision that is trauma-informed, emotionally responsive to the needs of the worker, and invites reflective practice leads to improvements for child protection workers and the children served by these systems (Hunt et al., 2016). It is argued that supervision may also increase resilience and act as a catalyst for PTG by helping child protection workers identify the impacts of the work and therefore start to process the work-related trauma. It, therefore, needs to be a priority in child protection workplaces for supervisors to be given appropriate training on how to supervise staff, particularly around supporting them with understanding trauma, the impacts of the work, and encouraging reflective practice (Radey & Stanley, 2018).

Conclusion

Child protection work is a high-risk occupation involving constant exposure to the trauma of others, coupled with difficult organizational factors including high workloads and turnover, and constant media and political scrutiny. Whilst individual practices are important in helping to reduce the impacts of work-related trauma, without a focus on changing the child protection systems to embed regular, supportive, and trauma-informed supervision, child protection systems are likely to remain in crisis. It is crucial that child protection agencies truly become trauma-informed services, acknowledging that all staff are open to being impacted by their work and actively embedding processes, such as supervision, to address this. In doing so, the potential for growth from work-related trauma inherent in child protection work may be increased. It is only through addressing the system issues characteristic of most child protection systems across the world that we can start to move towards workplaces that prioritize the wellbeing of their workers and the people the systems are meant to serve.

References

Auerbach, C., McGowan, B. G., Ausberger, A., Strolin-Goltzman, J., & Schudrich, W. (2010). Differential factors influencing public and voluntary child welfare workers' intention to leave. *Children and Youth Services Review, 32*(10), 1396–1402. doi:10.1016/j.childyouth.2010.06.008

Barrington, A., & Shakespeare-Finch, J. (2013). Posttraumatic Growth and Posttraumatic Depreciation as Predictors of Psychological Adjustment. *Journal of Loss and Trauma, 18,* 429-443. doi: 10.1080/15325024.2012.714210

Barth, R. P., Lloyd, E. C., Christ, S. L., Chapmen, M. V., & Dickinson, N. (2008). Child welfare worker characteristics and job satisfaction: A national study. *Social Work, 53,* 199–209. doi:10.1093/sw/53.3.199

Barto, B., Bartlett, J. D., Von Ende, A., Bodian, R., Norona, C. R., Griffin, J., Fraser, J. G., Kinniburgh, K., Spinazzola, J., Montagna, C., & Todd, M. (2018). The impact of a statewide trauma-informed child welfare initiative on children's permanency and maltreatment outcomes. *Child Abuse & Neglect, 81,* 149–160. doi:10.1016/j.chiabu.2018.04.023

Ben-Porat, A., Gottlieb, S., Refaeli, T., Shemesh, S., & Reuven Even Zahav, R. (2020). Vicarious growth among social work students: What makes the difference? *Health & Social Care in the Community, 28,* 662–669. doi:10.1111/hsc.12900

Braun, T. D., Uebelacker, L. A., Ward, M., Holzhauer, C. G., McCallister, K., & Abrantes, A. (2021). "We really need this": Trauma-informed yoga for Veteran women with a history of military sexual trauma. *Complementary Therapies in Medicine, 59.* doi:10.1016/j.ctim.2021.102729

Brockhouse, R., Msetfi, R. M., Cohen, K., & Joseph, S. (2011). Vicarious exposure to trauma and growth in therapists: The moderating effects of sense of coherence, organizational support, and empathy. *Journal of Traumatic Stress, 24,* 735–742. doi:10.1002/jts.20704

Carpenter, J., Webb, C. M., & Bostock, L. (2013). The surprisingly weak evidence base for supervision: Findings from a systematic review of research in child welfare practice (2000−2012). *Children and Youth Services Review, 35*, 1843−1853. doi:10.1016/j.childyouth.2013.08.014

Center for Advanced Studies in Child Welfare. (n.d.). *The Minnesota child welfare workforce stabilization study 2016: Child protection summary report.* http://cascw.umn.edu/wp-content/uploads/2016/09/WFSS_Summ ary.WEB_.pdf

Chenot, D. (2011). The vicious cycle: Recurrent interactions among the media, politicians, the public, and child welfare services organizations. *Journal of Public Child Welfare, 5*, 167−184. doi:10.1080/ 15548732.2011.566752

Chung, Y., & Choo, H. (2019). A structural path to job satisfaction, burnout, and intent to leave among child protection workers: A South Korean study. *Children and Youth Services Review, 100*, 304−312. doi:10.1016/j.childyouth.2019.03.018

Collins-Camargo, C., & Antle, B. (2018). Child welfare supervision: Special issues related to trauma-informed care in a unique environment. *The Clinical Supervisor, 37*, 64−82. doi:10.1080/07325223.2017.1382412

Connell, C. M., Lang, J. M., Zorba, B., & Stevens, K. (2019). Enhancing capacity for trauma-informed care in child welfare: Impact of a statewide systems change initiative. *American Journal of Community Psychology, 64*(3−4), 467−480. doi:10.1002/ajcp.12375

Conrad, D., & Kellar-Guenther, Y. (2006). Compassion fatigue, burnout, and compassion satisfaction among Colorado child protection workers. *Child Abuse & Neglect, 30*, 1071−1080.

Crews, D. A., Stolz-Newton, M., & Grant, N. S. (2016) The use of yoga to build self-compassion as a healing method for survivors of sexual violence. *Journal of Religion & Spirituality in Social Work: Social Thought, 35*,139−156. doi:10.1080/15426432.2015.1067583

Ellett, A. J., Ellis, J. I., Westbrook, T. M., & Dews, D. (2007). A qualitative study of 369 child welfare professionals' perspectives about factors contributing to employee retention and turnover. *Children and Youth Services Review, 29*, 264−281. doi:10.1016/j.childyouth.2006.07.005

Ferguson, S. M. (2006). Resolution of role conflict in public child welfare supervision. ProQuest Dissertations Publishing.

Gibbs, J. A. (2001). Maintaining front-line workers in child protection: A case for refocusing supervision. *Child Abuse Review, 10*, 323−335. doi:10.1002/car.707

Gladden, J., Morrow, R., & Climie, K. (2022). Trauma-sensitive yoga as an adjunctive treatment: The G.R.A.C.E. Model. *Journal of Creativity in Mental Health, 17*, 363−373. doi:10.1080/15401383.2021.1903373

Goddard, C., & Hunt, s. (2011). The complexities of caring for child protection workers: the contexts of practice and supervision. *Journal of Social Work Practice, 25*, 413−432. doi.org/10.1080/02650533.2011.626644

Hunt, S., Goddard, C., Cooper, J., Littlechild, B., & Wild, J. (2016). 'If I feel like this, how does the child feel?' Child protection workers, supervision, management, and organizational responses to parental violence. *Journal of Social Work Practice, 30,* 5–24. doi:10.1080/02650533.2015.1073145

Itzhaky, H., & Aviad-Hiebloom, A. (1998). How supervision and role stress in social work affect burnout. *Arete-Columbia South Carolina-, 22,* 29–43

Jacquet, S. E., Clark, S. J., Morazes, J. L., & Withers, R. (2008). The role of supervision in the retention of public child welfare workers. *Journal of Public Child Welfare, 1,* 27–54. doi:10.1300/J479v01n03_03

Jirek, S. L. (2015). Soul Pain: The hidden toll of working with survivors of physical and sexual violence. *SAGE Open, 5.* doi:10.1177/2158244015597905

Kelly, U., Haywood, T., Segell, E., & Higgins, M. (2021). Trauma-sensitive yoga for Post-Traumatic Stress Disorder in women veterans who experienced military sexual trauma: Interim results from a randomized controlled trial. *The Journal of Alternative and Complementary Medicine, 27,* S45–S59. doi:10.1089/acm.2020.0417

Kim, H., & Kao, D. (2014). A meta-analysis of turnover intention predictors among U.S. child welfare Workers. *Children and Youth Services Review, 47,* 214–223. doi:10.1016/j.childyouth.2014.09.015

Kinman, G., & Grant, L. (2011). Exploring stress resilience in trainee social workers: the role of emotional and social competencies. *The British Journal of Social Work, 41,* 261–275. doi:10.1093/bjsw/bcq088

Kong, G. S. (2005). Factors associated with turnover intention of Korean child protection workers. *Journal of the Korean Society of Child Welfare, 19,* 7–35

Lamothe, J., Couvrette, A., Lebrun, G., Yale-Souliè, G., Roy, C., Guay, S., & Geoffrion, S. (2018). Violence against child protection workers: A study of workers experiences, attributions, and coping strategies. *Child Abuse & Neglect, 81,* 308–321. doi:10.1016/j.chiabu.2018.04.027

Lang, J. K., Campbell, K., Shanley, P., Crusto, C. A., & Connell, C. M. (2016). Building capacity for trauma-informed care in the child welfare system: Initial results of a statewide implementations. *Child Maltreatment, 21,* 113–124. doi:10.1177/1077559516635273

Lietz, C., & Rounds, T. (2009). Strengths-based supervision: A child welfare supervision training project. *The Clinical Supervisor, 28,* 124–140. doi:10.1080/07325220903334065

Macy, R. J., Jones, E., Graham, L. M., & Roach, L. (2015). Yoga for trauma and related mental health problems: A meta-review with clinical and service recommendations. *Trauma, Violence, & Abuse, 19,* 1–23. doi:10.1177/1524838015620834

Manning-Jones, S., De Terte, I., & Stephens, C. (2016). Secondary traumatic stress, vicarious posttraumatic growth, and coping among health professionals; a comparison study. *New Zealand Journal of Psychology (Online), 45*, 20–29

Manning-Jones, S., de Terte, I., & Stephens, C. (2015). Vicarious post-traumatic growth: A systematic literature review. *International Journal of Wellbeing, 5*, 125–139. doi:10.5502/ijw.v5i2.8

McFadden, P., Mallett, J., & Leiter, M. (2018). Extending the two-process model of burnout in child protection workers: The role of resilience in mediating burnout via organizational factors of control, values, fairness, reward, workload, and community relationships. *Stress and Health, 34*, 72–83. doi:10.1002/smi.2763

McFadden, P., Campbell, A., & Taylor, B. (2015). Resilience and burnout in Child Protection Social Work: Individual and organisational themes from a systematic literature review. *The British Journal of Social Work, 45*, 1546–1563. doi:10.1093/bjsw/bct210

McFadden, P. (2020). Two sides of one coin? Relationships build resilience or contribute to burnout in child protection social work: Shared perspectives from Leavers and Stayers in Northern Ireland. *International Social Work, 63*, 164–176. doi:10.1177/0020872818788393

Mor Barak, M. E., Travis, D. J., Pyun, H., & Xie, B. (2009). The impact of supervision on worker outcomes: A meta-analysis. *Social Service Review, 83*, 3–32

Munro, E. (2011, April). The Munro Review of Child Protection Progress report: Moving towards a child centred system. National Child Welfare Workforce Institute. *Child welfare workforce demographics (2000-2010): Snapshot of the frontline child welfare caseworker.* https://ncwwi.org/files/Workforce_Demographic_Trends_May2011.pdf

Ong, I., Cashwell, C. S., & Downs, H. A. (2019). Trauma-sensitive yoga: A collective case study of women's trauma recovery from intimate partner violence. *Counseling Outcome Research and Evaluation, 10*, 19–33. doi:10.1080/21501378.2018.1521698

Pascoe, M. C., & Bauer, I. E. (2015). A systematic review of randomised control trials on the effects of yoga on stress measures and mood. *Journal of Psychiatric Research, 68*, 270–282. doi:10.1016/j.jpsychires.2015.07.013

Radey, M., & Stanley, L. (2018). "Hands on" versus "empty": Supervision experiences of frontline child welfare workers. *Children and Youth Services Review, 91*, 128–136. doi:10.1016/j.childyouth.2018.05.037

Regehr, C., Hemsworth, D., Leslie, B., Howe, P., & Chau, S. (2004). Predictors of post-traumatic distress in child welfare workers: a linear structural equation model. *Children and Youth Services Review, 26*, 331–346. doi:10.1016/j.childyouth.2004.02.003

Rhodes, A., Spinazzola, J., & van der Kolk, B. (2016). Yoga for adult women with chronic PTSD: A long-term follow-up study. *The Journal of Alternative and Complementary Medicine, 22*, 189–196. doi:10.1089/acm.2014.0407

Rutter, M. (1990) Psychosocial Resilience and Protective Mechanisms. In J. Rolf, A. S. Masten, D. Cicchetti, K. H. Nuechterlein, and S. Weintraub

(Eds.) *Risk and Protective Factors in the Development of Psychopathology*, pp. 181–214. Cambridge University Press.

Sharma, M. (2014). Yoga as an alternative and complementary approach for stress management: A systematic review. *Journal of Evidence-Based Complementary & Alternative Medicine, 19*, 59–67. doi:10.1177/2156587213503344

Stanley, J., Goddard, C., & Sanders, R. (2002). In the firing line: Violence and power in Child Protection Work. *Child & Family Social Work, 7*(4), 323–324. doi:10.1046/j.1365-206.2002.00258.x

Strolin-Goltzman, J., Kollar, S., & Trinkle, J. (2010). Listening to the voices of children in foster care: Youths speak out about child welfare workforce turnover and selection. *Social Work, 55*, 47–53. doi:10.1093/sw/55.1.47

Taylor, J., McLean, L., Korner, A., Stratton, E., & Glozier, N. (2020) Mindfulness and yoga for psychological trauma: systematic review and meta-analysis. *Journal of Trauma & Dissociation, 21*, 536–573. doi:10.1080/15299732.2020.1760167

Truter, E., Theron, L., & Fouché, A. (2018). No strangers to adversity: Resilience-promoting practices among South African women child protection social workers. *Qualitative Social Work, 17*, 712–731. doi:10.1177/14733 25016 688370

Um, M., & Harrison, D. F. (1998). Role stressors, burnout, mediators, and job satisfaction: A stress-strain-outcome model and empirical test. *Social Work Research, 22*, 100–115. doi:10.1093/swr/22.2.100

van der Kolk, B. (2014). *The body keeps the score: Mind, brain and body in the transformation of trauma*. U.K.: Penguin Random House.

Yi, L., Lian, Y., Ma, N., & Duan, N. (2022). A randomized controlled trial of the influence of yoga for women with symptoms of post-traumatic stress disorder. *Journal of Translational Medicine, 20*, 162. doi:10.1186/s12967-022-03356-0

Mental Health Workers

Louise Munro

13

*This chapter uses the term "mental health setting" for any workplace where the primary focus of the work is based on counseling, treatment, and/or interventions for people accessing mental health services. Workers in these settings are likely to spend a considerable amount of time building therapeutic relationships and participating in conversations about traumatic life experiences.

Chris

Chris works full-time in a counseling role and has recently started feeling a lack of enthusiasm for the work. At the end of the day, Chris looks at the caseload for the next day and starts to wonder whether the work is making any difference at all. Nonetheless, Chris stays back late reading files to prepare. One of the new clients has disclosed currently being in an abusive relationship. Chris ended a relationship with an abusive partner two years ago and this client's story resonates strongly. Chris has mentioned this in supervision and has been advised to refer on to a different worker, but having experience personally with this kind of situation is making it hard to let go of this client.

In the car on the way home, a news story reports on institutional child sex abuse, followed by a report on a local community that was devastated by recent flooding. Chris starts to wonder how much improvement is even possible in a world where there is so much bad news happening. At home, Chris' partner laments another evening spent arguing over getting home late, and even though the issue is quickly resolved, the effects of the argument hang around. Chris admits to becoming easily upset and aggravated over minor issues.

The next day Chris sees a client who unexpectedly reports a success story that points to the development of a new personal narrative that they've been working on collaboratively to navigate particular trauma triggers and achieve a previously unattainable goal. This experience has Chris feeling uplifted for the first time in

DOI: 10.4324/9781003292807-15

months and has Chris wondering if it's possible to engage more pur-
posefully with evidence of clients' experiences of success, resilience,
and triumph.

Introduction

This vignette hints at some well-known risks for therapists such as
burnout, countertransference, and the term "vicarious trauma" (McCann
& Pearlman, 1990). Chris' story will be familiar to many professionals
working in mental health settings. Chris could be a psychologist, psychiatrist, counselor, psychotherapist, social worker, nurse, or any kind of
worker whose role is to listen to clients retell their experiences of traumatic life events. In recent times these workers have been encouraged
to listen differently, for more than just symptoms but also for the
broader content and context that can be uncovered in clients' stories.
The paradigmatic shift in focus from "what's wrong with you" to "what
happened to you" has made much broader conversations, treatments, and
interventions possible (Sweeney et al., 2018).

Workers like Chris bear witness to stories of trauma for hours at a
time, day after day. Often called "the cost of caring" (Figley, 1995), these
negative effects can be pervasive, impacting workers physically, psychologically, emotionally, and in family and social relationships. The cost of
caring in the vignette is that Chris gets home from work exhausted and
short-tempered wondering about the value of the work and feeling negative about the future. Chris could also be showing signs of compassion
fatigue in questioning the meaning and usefulness of the work, and negative countertransference and/or burnout could explain staying back late
reviewing client files. Taken together, over time and given the tensions
that are spilling into personal relationships, Chris might be experiencing
vicarious trauma.

Chris' personal experience of trauma in an abusive relationship might
also have Chris feeling a strong pull to rescue or fix this client's situation. The conscious use of self in therapy can make for a rich and genuinely empathic therapeutic relationship, but it can also be triggering
and contribute to rescuing, unhelpful countertransference, burnout, and
over-identification. This risk is not just present for therapists, indeed
the experience of trauma is so widespread that social media platform
users are now routinely flagging the potential that a post with sensitive
or confronting information may be triggering, particularly for people
with trauma histories. In recognition of the unpredictable and individual
nature of what might be triggering content, the label "content warning"
is regularly appearing on social media (Charles et al., 2022). But what
happens to workers like Chris who don't get a trigger warning, and yet
need to be prepared to hear all types of traumatic content? Emotional

identification with a client is always a possibility and clients don't come with trigger warnings.

Despite decades of research into the health and wellbeing of mental health professionals, the terms burnout, compassion fatigue, counter-transference, and vicarious trauma have considerable overlap and are still used inconsistently and sometimes interchangeably. This lack of consistency is seen as an impediment to the prevention of the negative impacts of trauma work and the enhancement of clinical practice (Branson, 2019; Velasco et al., 2022). This chapter proposes that a focus on vicarious post-traumatic growth could move past these definitional issues and provide opportunities for improved worker health in mental health settings.

The Cost of Caring for Mental Health Professionals

The negative effects of trauma work on mental health professionals are well documented in a range of work settings including substance abuse centers (Cosden et al., 2016), complex psychological trauma services (Coleman et al., 2021), refugee support (Barrington & Shakespeare-Finch, 2013), sexual violence services (Crivatu et al., 2021), and many generic mental health services where trauma conversations occur.

A recent systemic review and meta-analysis of 52 research papers and over 10,000 participants in mental health and service settings explored the effects of occupational exposure to trauma (Velasco et al., 2022). The study investigated a range of variables including organizational factors, training level, therapist variables, theoretical orientation, lived experience, and personal characteristics. They found that the prevalence of posttraumatic stress disorder (PTSD) among mental health professionals was closer to the percentages found in clinical samples. At the same time, this study was unable to draw conclusions about risk factors but recommended that training for mental health professionals should cover compassion fatigue, vicarious trauma, and secondary trauma with an emphasis on normalizing these experiences to decrease negative stigmatization. At the end of this comprehensive review, the authors suggested that inconsistencies in methodologies and conceptual overlap hindered solid conclusions on the psychological effects of professional exposure to trauma.

Despite the inconsistencies in both the methods and the operationalization of key terms, there are a number of useful studies that demonstrate rigor. The impacts of caseload volume and diversity, peer support, access to training, organizational culture, and clinical supervision are commonly associated with negative outcomes for mental health professionals (Laverdière et al., 2019; Sutton et al., 2022). In short, there is broad agreement that both organizational interventions and individual actions can serve as protective factors and also contribute to vPTG (Barnhill et al., 2019; Cohen & Collens, 2013; Deaton et al., 2022; Knight, 2019; Sutton et al., 2022).

Posttraumatic Growth for Mental Health Professionals

Mental health professionals strive for their work to have a positive impact on clients. Professional development activities, peer and individual supervision, research, reading, exposure to new ideas, new therapies, and training, are all undertaken in an effort to relieve suffering and witness improvements in clients' lives. Much less time is spent exploring how, in a reciprocal sense, this therapy work might also have a positive impact on the lives of mental health professionals.

Interest in the positive effects of mental health work on workers is growing but the research is sparse. The 2005 landmark study by Arnold and colleagues was the first in-depth research into the potential for the positive effects of trauma work. This study found that descriptions of the positive effects of indirect exposure to trauma for workers were similar to the descriptions of PTG described by clients, prompting the use of the term vicarious posttraumatic growth (vPTG).

Historically, large swathes of mental health research are focused on symptom reduction for clients and on protective factors for workers. But this emphasis on measuring distress takes the research attention away from more eudemonic outcomes and presents a false dichotomy where distress and eudemonia are mutually exclusive or at best, separate pursuits. In contrast to the focus on symptom reduction/alleviation, research into PTG asserts distress can *be used* to foster PTG (Tedeschi et al., 2018). In the vignette, Chris feels uplifted when hearing of the client's success and starts to wonder how to intentionally listen for change and growth. The next section explores how therapeutic models shape what professionals are trained to notice and presents some of the strengths and limitations of particular practices and research designs in the context of encouraging PTG in clients and consequently in mental health professionals.

Finding What We Look For

Counseling and psychology research determines that best practice for the treatment of clients is based on symptom reduction/alleviation, and this generally provides evidence for efficacy using rigorous scientific research designs (Wampold & Imel, 2015). Consequently, randomized controlled trials find that cognitive behavioral therapies (CBT) (with or without adjustments to be "trauma-informed") meet the criteria for "best practice" and are often the first line of interventions promoted by peak professional bodies worldwide (see Watkins et al., 2018). But are these approaches the best practice for posttraumatic growth?

Manualized treatments like CBT lend themselves to the scientific model for research (Wampold & Imel, 2015) because these approaches are uniform, delivered in "doses" and have a list of specific ingredients (interventions) that are objectively identifiable and administered as per protocol. In contrast, evidence for non-manualized, collaborative, human-istic, and constructionist therapies is harder to establish and yet, they might provide more opportunities for clients to move beyond symptom alleviation and into the terrain for posttraumatic growth. Randomized controlled trials require the strict control of variables, and therapies that are not manualized can't be uniformly delivered as a protocol (Wampold & Imel, 2015). Furthermore, human emotions are not easily reduced and compartmentalized to suit research models and scientific methods that focus on symptom measurement to assess treatment.

Judith Herman, in the seminal work Trauma and Recovery (2015), makes this point and she goes on to discuss support for a range of approaches including what she has dubbed "plain old therapy" akin to the talking, relationship-based work of Carl Rogers. Linley and Joseph (2007) found that therapists using humanistic and transpersonal psycho-therapy reported more personal growth and change as a result of their professional work. They suggest this is because these orientations expli-citly acknowledge the role of suffering as an opportunity for growth. The aphorism "you find what you look for" is relevant. The next section of this chapter is a response to the question, what does my work practice have me looking for? How can I make visible inclusive, less pathologizing conceptualizations, life-affirming stories, and empowering narratives and understandings in my clients and consequently, myself?

Theoretical Opportunities

The sparse research in this space is clear that witnessing PTG in clients can foster the opportunity for vPTG in mental health workers (Arnold et al., 2005; Hyatt-Burkhart, 2014). Given this, some questions to con-sider when reflecting on practice are whether a chosen theoretical orien-tation makes visible an appreciation of the human spirit, capacity for growth and change, and the role of suffering in human development and meaning-making. Stuhlmille & Dunning (2000) caution against the emphasis on pathogenic diagnostic frameworks and encouraged a shift towards salutogenic models of post-trauma intervention. Two decades later there are still large gaps in the research into operationalizing salutogenic therapeutic interventions and their outcomes, with much of the focus on CBT training and research despite little support for the superiority of this approach.

In their groundbreaking work *The Great Psychotherapy Debate*, Wampold and Imel review decades of research, concluding that "the efficacy of psy-chotherapy now has been firmly established and is no longer a subject of debate" (2015, p. 32). Theories about the superiority of therapeutic orientations have faded in favor of the recognition that successful therapy is better explained by a combination of factors that are common to most therapies (Asay & Lambert, 1999; Wampold & Imel, 2015). Widely referred to as the "common factors theory" the research demonstrates that the bulk of client outcomes are explained by a combination of three key factors: the quality of the therapeutic alliance, the theoretical model, and the role of hope (variously explained as expectancy and allegiance) (Wampold & Imel, 2015).

Trauma-informed practice guidelines align with these factors in privileging safety and trust in the therapeutic relationship and acknowledging the role of hope (Herman, 2015). The role of hope, beliefs about the human condition, and change mechanisms are embedded in the philosophical underpinnings of all therapeutic approaches but they may be less visible and less accessible in models that focus on symptoms. Turning attention toward how therapeutic work generates hope and provides an audience for change bears examination if the focus is to foster PTG in clients.

With the current shift towards integrating therapeutic approaches, it is timely to consider how practice approaches might foster opportunities for witnessing PTG in clients and consequently foster vPTG. Wampold & Imel's (2015) extensive work on dispelling myths about the superiority of particular models of therapy also proposes that better outcomes have less to do with therapist experience and more to do with client feedback, the quality of the therapeutic alliance, and the capacity to adjust and individualize treatment rather than stick with a strict manualized approach.

Consistent with this trend, Tedeschi and Moore (2021) suggest the integration of cognitive-behavioral, narrative therapies, interpersonal and existential therapies as a PTG-based intervention model. Evidence-based approaches such as CBT and eye movement desensitization and reprocessing (EMDR) may not, on their own, attend to existential, narrative, and socio-political impacts for clients, a position also taken by Herman (2015). The model they suggest integrates therapeutic techniques that move beyond symptom reduction and incorporate key components of PTG that emphasize meaning-making, exploration of socio-cultural understandings, and the construction of new personal and interpersonal narratives. Systemic therapies, family therapies, and narrative therapies all explicitly invite clients to explore the layers of meaning that are created, re-created, and deconstructed in dialogical approaches and they support the action of effortful meaning-making.

In presenting the narrative element of the proposed integrative approach Tedeschi and Moore refer to "narrative therapies" in a general sense, while also citing evidence for narrative exposure therapy (NET) in working with refugees. However, narrative therapy (White & Epston, 1990) as a post-structural, non-manualized, social constructionist approach, is a world apart from NET, which has a behavioral basis and a manualized delivery. The existential element proposed by Tedeschi and Moore refers to our very human need to have meaning and purpose and make sense of our roles in relation to things we can and can't control, such as experiences of justice, fairness, and the impact of socio-cultural structures. Narrative therapy, based on the work of Michael White and David Epston, explicitly caters to many of these narrative *and* existential elements by making room in conversations for political, philosophical, and narrative deconstructions.

There is a growing appreciation for the integration of approaches in counseling and psychotherapy, but the process of integration is not straightforward and very little has been written on how to integrate across epistemological positions. Dickerson (2010) offers a useful analysis of the possibilities and impediments to integration with an emphasis on intentional reflective practice and a deconstruction of underlying philosophical assumptions that are embedded in theoretical orientations. She argues that there are epistemological incongruencies that prohibit coherent integration at a philosophical level. For example, where one theoretical orientation might privilege the co-construction of meaning in a relational dialogue between client and therapist, another model may privilege a textbook definition that requires a specific intervention.

Denborough (2019) explores this in-depth when raising the question of how neuroscience (a structural, scientific epistemology) engages with narrative therapy (a distinctly post-structural and social-constructionist epistemology). Acknowledging that neuroscience and neuropsychotherapy feature prominently in the trauma-informed discourse and that narrative therapy offers possibilities for effortful meaning-making that incorporates socio-political contexts, Denborough's discussion paper makes an important contribution to thinking about integrating seemingly incompatible epistemologies.

Chris reflects on the therapy model the workplace has endorsed and realizes that it doesn't really invite conversations with the client about meaning-making practices or the deconstruction of the political context that contributes to the experience of trauma. Bringing these reflections to supervision with peers and with the clinical supervisor could offer some insights into how other professionals are integrating therapies and accessing professional development to extend their therapeutic skills and understanding of more salutogenic models.

If it is that the mental health field is to genuinely encourage a salutogenic model for workers and clients then the field will benefit from increased attention to mixed-methods and qualitative research methods. Psychology and counseling have made great strides in creating valid and reliable measures of symptoms, however, PTG is evidenced in stories as well as, and potentially more so, than numbers. The question "what's wrong with you?" is an invitation to list symptoms and this creates an almost irresistible invitation to measure them. In contrast, "what happened to you?" is an invitation to engage in storying.

> So pervasive is this human predilection toward 'storying' experience that our species might appropriately be labeled not simply homo sapiens, emphasizing our effort to seek knowledge, but more

specifically homo narrans stressing our tendency to organize such knowledge in storied form.

(Neimeyer, 2004, p. 53)

As therapeutic work adopts a more integrative approach there is room for research to follow this lead and integrate qualitative and quantitative methods. Although there is a lot of published mixed-methods research, the dominance of quantitative findings and the goal of generalizability diminishes the potential reach of rigorous qualitative research. Like therapy integration, there are complex epistemological considerations in order to rigorously undertake qualitative research and then integrate qualitative and quantitative research which have substantially different epistemological bases (see Levitt et al., 2021).

Workplace Opportunities for vPTG

In a review of the literature on therapist resilience Hou and Skovholt (2020) identified a range of risk factors for therapists including caseload, work hours, availability of supervision, and level of trauma-related client exposure. Careful attention to these factors is important in mitigating burnout (Barnhill et al., 2019). Proactive measures are also encouraged. Hou and Skovholt (2020) identify some of the basics that are often forgotten when stress mounts, such as healthy eating, sleep, exercise, actively coping with stress rather than ignoring it, and engaging in regular supervision. In providing fertile ground for time, space, and reflection, Barnhill et al. (2019) specifically point to mindful practices like yoga, meditation, and tai chi to cultivate positive emotions such as appreciation, attention, and compassion, while also making a contribution to resilience. In concluding their qualitative research, Hou and Skovholt identified that "highly resilient therapists are (a) drawn to strong interpersonal relationships, (b) actively engage with self, (c) possess a core values and beliefs framework, and (d) desire to learn and grow" (2020, p. 386). These are also key individual qualities that are present in the characteristics of PTG (Tedeschi et al., 2018).

Workplace policies, procedures, and the culture of the work setting have a big impact on worker health and well-being. Just like clients in a therapeutic relationship, it is hard to imagine possibilities for vPTG without feeling valued, supported, and safe in the workplace. Decades of research shows that work-related factors are key contributors to burnout (O'Connor et al., 2018). In a review of the literature on organizational factors that contribute to vicarious trauma in mental health professionals, the authors found that it was imperative for organizations to acknowledge and validate the existence of secondary traumatic stress and they highlight "the importance of regular supervision within supportive supervisory relationships, strong peer support networks, and balanced and diverse caseloads" (Sutton et al., 2022, p. 1).

The value of "meaning-making" has been a consistent finding in research into PTG and vPTG and, understanding the importance of confidentiality, supervision is the most likely opportunity that therapists have to engage in meaning-making about their work. This opportunity will also depend on the kind of supervision a workplace offers. Long (2020) makes the point that supervision context is important and an emphasis on clinical problem-solving may leave little room for a focus on the impact of trauma stories on therapists. Knowing that "effortful meaning-making" has been identified as a facilitator of positive change for therapists (Barrington & Shakespeare-Finch, 2013), ensuring supervision provides for this type of focus and reflection is important.

However, not all models of supervision provide for this type of reflection. In a study with Australian trauma counselors working in a refugee service, one of the key findings was the lack of attention in supervision to socio-political context (Long, 2020). This finding is captured by a participant's response; "you go to work on a day when the government has made a decision that has an effect on the client population as a whole; that can be the thing that shatters perception and shocks the worker, not the client trauma" (Long, 2020, p. 114). This is a powerful reminder that none of us live in a vacuum and human responses to both trauma and trauma stories are situated in a social-political context that most therapeutic and supervision orientations make little attempt to deconstruct.

Taking the lead from Tedeschi and Moore's (2021) article on the integration of therapeutic orientations mentioned earlier in this chapter, there appears to be room for a similar approach to supervision orientations. Isomorphic models of supervision would propose that supervision should mirror the therapy being delivered. This provides an experience of the therapeutic orientation along with a demonstration of how the model can be delivered in the context of encouraging reflective practice (Lee & Nelson, 2022). This style of supervision is qualitatively different from the line management style of supervision where a superior or team leader delivers supervision in order to mitigate problems, focusing on worker competence, problem-solving, workload capacity, and caseload discussion (Lee & Nelson, 2022).

Reflective supervision and small group peer supervision can provide the essentials of validation, affirmation, meaning-making, safety, support, and trust. Sometimes it is not possible to get this kind of supervision in the workplace because there is a conflict of interest where a superior may also be tasked with evaluation and holds a level of power that might inhibit vulnerability for mental health workers. In these instances, peer supervision and individual supervision with external supervisors provide a necessary alternative.

Chris attends a small peer supervision group for mental health workers, outside of their workplaces, once every month. They use supervision to discuss clinical presentations and ethical dilemmas, but also to share their own success stories and explore their own responses, positive and negative, to client stories. They reflect on their intentions in the therapeutic space and their hopes for their clients and themselves and they connect these ideas to their own evolving world views and belief systems. Chris' mandatory workplace supervision focuses on outcome measures and compliance with ethical and legal guidelines which is really helpful, but this external supervision feels more supportive of the therapist as a person rather than the therapist as a worker.

Chris is supported by the group to refer a particular client to another therapist after recognizing some triggers from a past personal experience. Chris also decides to approach the team leader about workload issues and the risk of burnout. At the end of the session, the group does five minutes of mindfulness, focusing on breathing and bodily sensations, and consciously attending to tight areas of the body. The participants head home with a renewed sense of purpose in their work, gratitude for their life circumstances, and a deep appreciation for the people they share their lives with.

Conclusion

Vicarious posttraumatic growth for mental health professionals has been characterized by a focus on meaning-making, changes to world view, increased sense of professional competence, improved capacity for empathy, increased compassion, and a greater appreciation for life circumstances (Barrington & Shakespeare-Finch, 2014; Deaton et al., 2022; Knight, 2019; Michalchuk & Martin, 2019; Tedeschi et al., 2018).

> … simply acknowledging the possibility of vicarious posttraumatic growth could have important consequences for psychotherapists and their clients. Adopting a more inclusive, less pathologizing conceptualization (Greening, 2001; King, 2001) of trauma work—as an endeavour that holds the promise of life-affirming benefits as well as sadness and pain—might help clinicians to view themselves, their clients, and their work in new and empowering ways.
>
> (Arnold et al., 2005p. 260)

This chapter has presented an argument for increasing research and practice attention to opportunities for vPTG for mental health professionals. Trauma is widespread, and trauma work has the potential to both exhaust and uplift professionals. This chapter has presented four areas of attention that could foster more opportunities for vPTG: theoretical considerations, individual factors, organizational opportunities, and research suggestions. In closing, the vignette provides a scenario incorporating these opportunities and illustrating the possibilities for vPTG in mental health professionals.

References

Arnold, D., Calhoun, L. G., Tedeschi, R., & Cann, A. (2005). Vicarious posttraumatic growth in psychotherapy. *Journal of Humanistic Psychology, 45*, 239–263. doi:10.1177/0022167805274729

Asay, T. P., & Lambert, M. J. (1999). The empirical case for the common factors in therapy: Quantitative findings. *The Heart and Soul of Change: What Works in Therapy*, 23–55. doi:10.1037/11132-001

Barnhill, J., Fisher, J. W., Kimel-Scott, K., & Weil, A. (2019). Trauma-Informed Care: Helping the Healthcare Team Thrive. In M. R. Gerber (Ed.) *Trauma-Informed Healthcare Approaches: A Guide for Primary Care*, pp. 197–213. Springer International Publishing. doi:10.1007/978-3-030-04342-1_11

Barrington, A. J., & Shakespeare-Finch, J. (2013). Working with refugee survivors of torture and trauma: An opportunity for vicarious post-traumatic growth. *Counselling Psychology Quarterly, 26*, 89–105. doi:10.1080/09515070.2012.727553

Barrington, A. J., & Shakespeare-Finch, J. (2014). Giving voice to service providers who work with survivors of torture and trauma. *Qualitative Health Research, 24*, 1686–1699. doi:10.1177/1049732314549023

Branson, D. C. (2019). Vicarious trauma, themes in research, and terminology: A review of literature. *Traumatology, 25*, 2–10. doi:10.1037/trm0000161

Charles, A., Hare-Duke, L., Nudds, H., Franklin, D., Llewellyn-Beardsley, J., Rennick-Egglestone, S., Gust, O., Ng, F., Evans, E., Knox, E., Townsend, E., Yeo, C., & Slade, M. (2022). Typology of content warnings and trigger warnings: Systematic review. *PLOS ONE, 17*, e0266722. doi:10.1371/journal.pone.0266722

Cohen, K., & Collens, P. (2013). The impact of trauma work on trauma workers: A metasynthesis on vicarious trauma and vicarious post-traumatic growth. *Psychological Trauma, 5*, 570–580. doi:10.1037/a0030388

Coleman, A. M., Chouliara, Z., & Currie, K. (2021). Working in the field of complex psychological trauma: A framework for personal and professional, training, and supervision. *Journal of Interpersonal Violence, 36*, 2791–2815. doi:10.1177/0886260518759062

Cosden, M., Sanford, A., Koch, L. M., & Lepore, C. E. (2016). Vicarious trauma and vicarious posttraumatic growth among substance abuse treatment providers. *Substance Abuse, 37*, 619–624. doi:10.1080/08897077.2016.1181695

Crivatu, I. M., Horvath, M. A. H., & Massey, K. (2021). The Impacts of Working With Victims of Sexual Violence: A Rapid Evidence Assessment. *Trauma, Violence, & Abuse*, 15248380211016024. doi:10.1177/15248380211016024

Deaton, J. D., Ohrt, J. H., Linich, K., McCartney, E., & Glascoe, G. (2022). Vicarious posttraumatic growth: A systematic review and thematic synthesis across helping professions. *Traumatology, 29*, 17–26. doi:10.1037/trm0000375

Denborough, D. (2019). Travelling down the neuro-pathway: Narrative practice, neuroscience, bodies, emotions and the affective turn. *The International Journal of Narrative Therapy and Community Work.* https://www.semanticscholar.org/paper/Travelling-down-the-neuro-path way%3A-Narrative-a-nd-Denborough/973ef8bf93aac33c5c6e17f1c 0445f3e81c66865

Dickerson, V. C. (2010). Positioning oneself within an epistem-ology: Refining our thinking about integrative approaches. *Family Process, 49*, 349–368. doi:10.1111/j.1545-5300.2010.01327.x

Figley, C. R. (Ed.). (1995). *Compassion fatigue: Coping with secondary trau-matic stress disorder in those who treat the traumatized.* New York: Brunner/Mazel

Herman, J. (2015). *Trauma and recovery: The aftermath of violence from domestic abuse to political terror* (1R edition). Basic Books

Hou, J. M., & Skovholt, T. M. (2020). Characteristics of highly resilient therapists. *Journal of Counseling Psychology, 67*, 386–400. doi:10.1037/cou0000401

Hyatt-Burkhart, D. (2014). The experience of vicarious posttraumatic growth in mental health workers. *Journal of Loss and Trauma, 19*, 452–461. doi:10.1080/15325024.2013.797268

Knight, C. (2019). Trauma informed practice and care: Implications for field instruction. *Clinical Social Work Journal, 47*, 79–89. doi:10.1007/s10615-018-0661-x

Laverdière, O., Kealy, D., Ogrodniczuk, J. S., Chamberland, S., & Descôteaux, J. (2019). Psychotherapists' Professional Quality of Life. *Traumatology (Tallahassee, Fla.), 25*, 208–215. doi:10.1037/trm0000177

Lee, R. E., & Nelson, T. (2022). *The contemporary relational supervisor* (Second edition). Routledge, Taylor & Francis Group

Levitt, H. M., Morrill, Z., Collins, K. M., & Rizo, J. L. (2021). The meth-odological integrity of critical qualitative research: Principles to support design and research review. *Journal of Counseling Psychology, 68*, 357–370. doi:10.1037/cou0000523

Linley, P. A., & Joseph, S. (2007). Therapy work and therapists' positive and negative well-being. *Journal of Social and Clinical Psychology, 26*, 385–403. doi:10.1521/jscp.2007.26.3.385

Long, S. (2020). Supervisors' perception of vicarious trauma and growth in Australian refugee trauma counsellors. *Australian Social Work, 73*, 105–117. doi:10.1080/0312407X.2018.1501587

McCann, I. L., & Pearlman, L. A. (1990). Vicarious traumatization: A framework for understanding the psychological effects of working with victims. *Journal of Traumatic Stress, 3*, 131–149. doi:10.1007/BF00975140

Michalchuk, S., & Martin, S. L. (2019). Vicarious resilience and growth in psychologists who work with trauma survivors: An interpretive phenomenological analysis. *Professional Psychology: Research and Practice, 50*, 145–154. doi:10.1037/pro0000212

Neimeyer, R. A. (2004). Fostering Posttraumatic Growth: A Narrative Elaboration. *Psychological Inquiry, 15*, 53–59. JSTOR

O'Connor, K., Neff, D. M., & Pitman, S. (2018). Burnout in mental health professionals: A systematic review and meta-analysis of prevalence and determinants. *European Psychiatry, 53*, 74–99. doi:10.1016/j.eurpsy.2018.06.003

Stuhlmiller, C., & Dunning, C. (2000). Challenging the mainstream: From pathogenic to salutogenic models of posttrauma intervention. In J. M. Violanti, D. Paton, & C. Dunning (Eds.) *Posttraumatic stress intervention: Challenges, issues, and perspectives* (pp. 10–42). Charles C Thomas Publisher

Sutton, L., Rowe, S., Hammerton, G., & Billings, J. (2022). The contribution of organisational factors to vicarious trauma in mental health professionals: A systematic review and narrative synthesis. *European Journal of Psychotraumatology, 13*, 1–21. doi:10.1080/20008198.2021.2022278

Sweeney, A., Filson, B., Kennedy, A., Collinson, L., & Gillard, S. (2018). A paradigm shift: relationships in trauma-informed mental health services. *BJPsych Advances, 24*, 319–333. doi:10.1192/bja.2018.29

Tedeschi, R. G., & Moore, B. A. (2021). Posttraumatic growth as an integrative therapeutic philosophy. *Journal of Psychotherapy Integration, 31*, 180–194. doi:10.1037/int0000250

Tedeschi, R. G., Shakespeare-Finch, J., Taku, K., & Calhoun, L. G. (2018). *Posttraumatic Growth: Theory, Research and Applications.* Routledge

Velasco, J., Sanmartín, F. J., Gálvez-Lara, M., Cuadrado, F., & Moriana, J. A. (2022). Psychological Effects of Professional Exposure to Trauma and Human Suffering: Systematic Review and Meta-Analysis. *Trauma, Violence, & Abuse*, 15248380221074314. doi:10.1177/15248380221074314

Wampold, B. E., & Imel, Z. E. (2015). *The Great Psychotherapy Debate: The Evidence for What Makes Psychotherapy Work* (2nd ed.). Routledge. doi:10.4324/9780203582015

Watkins, L. E., Sprang, K. R., & Rothbaum, B. O. (2018). Treating PTSD: A review of evidence-based psychotherapy interventions. *Frontiers in Behavioral Neuroscience, 12*, 258. doi:10.3389/fnbeh.2018.00258

White, M., & Epston, D. (1990). *Narrative means to therapeutic ends.* W. W. Norton

Disaster Victim Identification Specialists

14

Peter Ellis and Howard Way

John

A terrorist bomb explodes in a central city hotel resulting in the collapse of the building and the death of many people in and around the hotel site. As the site is cleared and rendered safe, a team is tasked to retrieve and identify the dead. Included in that team are several young police officers and emergency workers, many of whom have no experience in the management of mass fatality incidents. Exposure to this site and the need to handle the damaged bodies causes distress to some who have never seen such human destruction. One of the officers, John, is recently bereaved following the death of his child due to sudden infant death syndrome. He is particularly distraught as there are several dead children who were in the small creche that was located in the destroyed building. The officers who work with John need to support and protect their fellow worker while maintaining maximum efficiency and accuracy during the whole identification process. This includes the handling of the human remains as well as the full scientific process which aims to establish identity and the collection of relevant important forensic evidence to aid in the criminal investigation. Support also needs to be provided both by and for the various scientific experts who participate in the identification process. These can include pathologists, anthropologists, odontologists, forensic biologists, and fingerprint experts as well as others not directly exposed to the actual human remains but who nevertheless may be constantly contacted by bereaved relatives enquiring after their lost loved ones.

Background

Incidents in which people die can and do occur at any time and place. These mass-fatality incidents may be the result of many and varied situations and include natural disasters such as earthquakes, bushfires, or tidal waves as well as unnatural incidents such as large transportation

DOI: 10.4324/9781003292807-16

accidents including aircraft and train crashes, collapsed buildings, and even the consequences of criminal activity such as multiple shooting events and explosions. While some of these incidents may be predicted in general terms, for example, major weather events, most occur without warning and any responses must be implemented without any effective preparation that could normally have been expected to reduce or minimize death and injury. Effectively, a disaster that leads to multiple fatalities is often accompanied by confusion, chaos, and disorganization that would inevitably follow an unexpected catastrophe.

Incidents in which many people die, especially those in which man-made or criminal activity has been a factor, produce a number of challenges for attending authorities. Given that such incidents will not necessarily result in the death of everyone involved, the rescue, support, and medical management of survivors and other injured persons will inevitably be the first and most important societal response. The effects that such an incident and its ensuing complications can have on attending workers are of great importance but are outside the scope of this chapter and covered in detail elsewhere in this text. Additionally, especially in those situations in which criminal activity is a possibility, or in which some accidental event has precipitated the incident, an urgent forensic investigation may be appropriate to address necessary investigative and forensic study. It is appropriate that after death the bodies of the deceased should be handled and disposed of in a safe and efficient manner all the time paying notice to relevant requirements, which may themselves vary depending on the needs of the immediate community. Such handling includes, and is indeed usually centered around, the identification of individual bodies and body parts and the return of those remains to their respective families. Subsequent disposal of the remains by families will vary depending on their appropriate culture or religion. The intense pressure to return deceased remains to families, whether political or societal, ensures that the identification process and subsequent handling of human remains should be conducted in as timely and efficient a method as possible. This very pressure may indeed add to the significant challenges faced by attending teams both from a procedural as well as a personal angle.

In recent history, many international communities, especially through security and policing agencies, have developed services to facilitate the recovery and identification of the dead after mass fatality incidents. These agencies are varied in their background, governance, staffing, and management, and those operatives who represent such agencies will possess wide-ranging policing, medical, paramedical, scientific, or parascientific skills. Additionally, the backgrounds of those responders faced with the involvement in the management of a mass-fatality incident can be so diverse that it will be very difficult for authorities to generalize policies whereby the personal support and supervision of such staff can be designed and instituted. For some, involvement in such a confronting incident may seem to be part of "normal" activity, such as specialist disaster recovery teams, whereas for others these incidents may present a dramatic, unique, and often confronting exercise in body management.

Considering the vignette scenario, John would not normally consider that he would be expected to be in the front-line responding team in view of his previous life experiences. Indeed, the disaster victim recovery teams should be assembled from groups of dedicated personnel who have not only volunteered to participate in this type of work but who have been screened and specifically trained for such work. Unfortunately, however, the scale and timing of these incidents are such that frequently insufficient numbers of trained personnel are available at short notice. Potentially vulnerable personnel such as John may therefore be unexpectedly recruited and exposed to personal and psychologically hazardous situations.

The location of such disasters can, of course, be very varied and it is therefore frequently a requirement for responders to travel from their normal or home location to a distant site. This may involve overseas travel or relocation to a relatively distant or remote part of their home country. This travel, especially when enforced with short notice, has the potential to increase the stress placed upon responders by causing them to work in an unfamiliar environment superimposed upon the technical or emotional stresses associated with the underlying disaster response. For example, in the aftermath of destruction brought on by severe weather such as a cyclone or typhoon, first responders may arrive at the site of the disaster and be faced with total devastation including loss of infrastructure, most means of effective communication, and even personal support. These conditions may persist for days or even weeks and responders who are responsible for the manual handling of human remains may be faced with the disfigurement or fragmentation of those remains. If the situation persists, especially in tropical conditions, decomposition of the remains may produce further disfigurement and presentation of the remains in an increasingly confronting manner.

Personnel who may be involved in the response to mass-fatality incidents can be many and varied. It is evident that initial responders may be emergency workers or from policing organizations, but it may also be true that scientific investigators including pathologists, odontologists and anthropologists may also be involved in this process. Additionally, other personnel who may be exposed to some unexpected side-effects of disaster response can include administrative staff who act as coordinators for some of the more "frontline" personnel, individuals tasked to perform "menial jobs" such as cleaners and body movers, and even those involved in the medicolegal investigation such as coroners and prosecutors and their staff. All these other personnel, as well as those more directly involved in identification and body handling, may potentially be exposed to very real psychological stresses by the whole process of death investigation.

Traditionally, the process of body identification after mass-fatality incidents has been classified into several phases, namely scene investigation, post-mortem body examination, and antemortem record investigation culminating in the reconciliation of post-mortem and antemortem information to result in the final identification of the remains. It is appropriate that each section of this process is addressed individually as the challenges and possible responses in respect of psychological personnel support vary according to the potential challenges facing the workers involved in each of the sections (Brondolo et al., 2012).

Scene Investigation

The scene of a mass-fatality incident can present a very confronting challenge to those workers tasked with addressing all the various issues, especially those specifically involved in handling and management of the dead (Cordner & Ellingham 2017). While the nature of such an incident can vary dramatically, the principal task of responders, assuming that management of the living has been addressed, is to ensure that the bodies, both intact and disfigured or fragmented, are handled respectfully but also efficiently as it is essential that any evidence that is needed to either identify those remains or to assist in the forensic investigation of the incident is preserved and retained. The varied nature of such disasters, together with their frequently remote location, means that the personnel frequently tasked to address these early issues may indeed be first responders who are untrained and unprepared to face the very real, intensely stressful, and confronting tasks and issues that inevitably constitute early disaster response. Even those personnel who are highly trained, such as police scene responders and scientific experts, may not be expecting the level of disruption often seen in major mass fatality events or the failure of infrastructure and services that can accompany mass disasters. The concept of self-care as well as the assistance of colleagues and authorities to prevent and manage disaster-related stress before it develops is well recognized but not always well implemented (Quevillon et al., 2016).

As indicated above, the management of a mass-fatality incident scene, once infrastructure issues and personal dangers have been addressed, relates to the careful examination and recording of each individual set of remains, whether those remains be whole intact bodies or damaged/fragmented pieces. These are carefully numbered, recorded, and prepared for collection in such a way that subsequent examination can be performed without creating any misleading or confusing evidence. Insofar as the potential exposure to personal stress or emotionally upsetting issues is concerned, whether the incident is of natural origin or of an unnatural or potentially criminal nature does not usually change the inherent dangers. Therefore, the responders must be prepared to face any potential confronting situation in respect of bodily disfigurement or damage. It is appropriate, therefore, that strategies and mechanisms for preventing the development of stress be instituted during the preparation and training process for staff and other personnel who may be called upon to respond to such incidents. It is well-known that the potential to develop acute stress disorder (ASD) or post-traumatic stress disorder (PTSD) can be increased in those staff whose duty it is to respond to such disasters, especially if worksite intervention strategies are not implemented or, at least, attempted (Brondolo et al., 2008).

It is, therefore, appropriate to attempt to institute a preventive interventional program for staff who may be exposed to such a situation. This will include persons in occupations who may be part of the first responses or scene examination, as well as those involved in body recovery work. This will often include police in the emergency response teams as well as relevant scientific experts such as pathologists, odontologists, anthropologists, forensic biologists, and fingerprint experts. Such a program would certainly include educational information about the effects of particular types of events as well as the potential health consequences of relevant exposure to physical and biological hazards and the inevitable size and nature of such a mass fatality incident. Technical drills that simulate such incidents allow first-response practitioners to train and prepare effective personal and group reactions to such mass disasters and their potential stress-inducing sequelae.

Finally, it is appropriate that all responding staff, regardless of background, should be supervised and managed throughout the ongoing deployment to the site of the disaster to ensure that any adverse effects, either physical or psychological, are avoided, minimized, or, if necessary, managed appropriately (Quevillon et al., 2016). The duration of such exposure will vary according to available resources and the size and location of the incident but can vary from a small number of days to several weeks and therefore personnel management, including appropriate rotation as well as post deployment care, should be carefully instituted.

In our vignette scenario, John found himself in a role for which he didn't volunteer, and his recent bereavement would have raised concern if it had been recorded during the screening process that should be conducted while assessing volunteers for suitability in this work. Such a bereavement would not inevitably disqualify an individual applying for such a role, but it would ensure that relevant and appropriate welfare support and monitoring were in place in the event of operational activation.

Postmortem Body Examination

The examination of human remains is usually conducted within a formal mortuary structure, and it is normal that appropriate facilities are provided to attending personnel, whether they be police or relevant scientific investigators. However, as well as those persons normally considered to be responsible for examining the human remains, other individuals may be exposed to the inevitably confronting nature of those remains that need to be studied, and it is appropriate that all supportive measures provided for and available to the scientific investigators should also be retained for those other persons who will also be exposed to the challenging sights. These may include those responsible for moving bodies and paramedical personnel as well as radiographers, cleaners, and administrative staff who are often forgotten in the context of the management of forensic personnel involved in a mass fatality incident response (Glaysher et al., 2016).

The phenomenon of secondary traumatic stress, burnout, and compassion satisfaction is well recognized among law enforcement and legal professionals as well as human service providers but has only recently been acknowledged to occur among forensic science operatives (Levin et al., 2021). Additionally, Levin et al. noted that field-based forensic science professionals, especially those involved in major incident responses, demonstrated higher levels of secondary traumatic stress compared to those professionals based in laboratories. Additionally, those individuals who believed that their organizations were addressing, or at least attempting to address, issues of stress and trauma seemed to demonstrate lower levels of secondary traumatic stress. This consideration reinforces the need for organizations employing or activating field-based professionals to acknowledge the issue of stress and trauma, especially in those situations where there is direct exposure to traumatic scenes or where there is direct contact with the families of victims.

It is relevant to acknowledge that this part of the identification process involves considerable handling of human remains, some of which may be considerably damaged or even fragmented. The process of postmortem examination involves movement of the human remains from the location of storage to the place of examination, possibly including radiological or some other supplementary study. The examination process itself is usually conducted by professional scientific operatives, such as pathologists, odontologists, forensic assistants, forensic biologists, or fingerprint specialists, although even for those experienced individuals the sheer scale of many of these operations may prove daunting and intimidating and may be a significant factor in precipitating adverse psychological responses. After the post-mortem examination process has been completed, the remains will usually be reconstructed in preparation for ultimate restoration to families and those remains are returned to the location of storage pending satisfactory completion of identification and/or legal and forensic investigative processes. It should also not be forgotten that there may be other persons attending these processes whose duties do not usually entail involvement with human remains and these may include police personnel who may be present as observers, document scribers, photographers, nursing staff, or other individuals, all of whom are consequently exposed to the potential for developing distressing exposure-related responses.

Antemortem Record Investigation

The process of identification of human remains involves the comparison of post-mortem observations with available antemortem information in the hope that sufficient identity exists between different categories of records, documented in each of these categories, to allow the identification of the individual to be completed and confirmed. This implies the very detailed collection of data and information relating to every individual, especially within those categories deemed to be unique, such as fingerprints, odontology, and forensic biology (Interpol, 2018). While the personnel involved in this aspect of the identification process are much less exposed to the confronting sights and smells that are associated with examination of human remains, they are potentially subjected to sensations that can be equally but more subtly distressing. In particular, the individuals tasked with consulting bereaved relatives can find this exposure quite daunting and the potential for creating adverse psychological responses within these investigators must be recognized by management and controlling authorities. In the vignette scenario, John would be particularly susceptible to succumbing to this situation and it would be very challenging to expect him to interact with families bereaved of children without expecting similar adverse personal effects. It is frequently recommended that counselors or similar supportive personnel accompany investigators who are seeking to collect antemortem information from bereaved relatives. These counselors are usually involved in the context of supporting families of presumed disaster victims although it must be recognized that investigators themselves should be considered as potentially exposed to vicarious bereavement distress. In the event that supporting counsellor staffing is not available, it is essential that the investigating team be provided with appropriate psychological support. This support may include formal psychological preparation as well as peer-to-peer support and cooperation, and the encouragement of social interaction and professional/counsellor assistance (Brooks et al., 2015).

Reconciliation

After the post-mortem (PM) examination has been completed and all the PM information collected and documented, it is necessary to compare that information with antemortem (AM) data recorded on known individuals. Finding identical information on the various AM and PM data records especially within the primary identifying categories permits the legal authority to assign a specific identity to those human remains. That allows those remains to be formally identified and, depending on the legal circumstances, permits the release of the remains and their return to the families or appropriate community. While this is essentially a legalistic process which should not involve much exposure to the human remains, except in those situations where re-examination is required for specific reasons, the potential to precipitate further emotional stress on operating individuals, while not great, should not be ignored. It is known, for example, that considerable external pressure may be applied by community or political influences, and this can produce quite a stressful environment during which the reconciliation process must be undertaken. It is, therefore, appropriate for the employing authority to ensure that staff involved in this reconciliation process are permitted to operate without excess external pressures and with full institutional support.

Long-Term Effects

Finally, when the immediate mass fatality incident has been addressed and all forensic and identification procedures completed, it should not be forgotten that there may indeed be quite long-term effects for many operational staff. It is known that there are potential risk factors for significant psychological distress including the development of post-traumatic stress among those disaster workers some time after the incident in which they were working has been apparently finalized (Sakuma et al., 2015, Nagamine et al., 2016). It is appropriate that long-term health outcomes among disaster and humanitarian responders are managed by appropriate surveillance, risk mitigation, and relevant management. There is considerable literature reporting this as an issue although it should be noted that there is no specific recommended response that would address all potential situations (Garbern et al., 2016).

Strategies for Managing Adverse Effects on Forensic Responders to Mass Fatality Incidents

Brondolo et al. (2008) have suggested some ways of minimizing and addressing the development of adverse after-effects in forensic workers responding to mass fatality incidents. It must, however, be acknowledged that not all changes in MFI responders are negative. Indeed, the concept of posttraumatic growth is gaining increasing recognition and should be recognized as a very real positive outcome among some responders to mass fatality incidents (Tedeschi et al., 2018). The close interaction of these responders with bereaved families, and in particular the ability to assist such families to recover from these disasters and gain closure, can be very fulfilling for emergency workers and especially those who are tasked with direct personal interaction with relatives of the dead. For example, in the vignette scenario, if John were part of the team responsible for interacting with families of the deceased children, it is quite possible that his own personal experiences from losing a child could be used positively to support the bereaved families but also to give him strength in counteracting the personal grief that such a challenging scenario would inevitably precipitate both in the families as well as in himself.

At an institutional level, post-traumatic growth is being increasingly recognized as one of the possible results of the involvement of disaster responders to such apparently traumatic situations (Leppma et al., 2018). In this study, police officers working in the New Orleans area following Hurricane Katrina were assessed and it was noted that those who were regularly at risk of trauma exposure were more likely to benefit from the social support and higher levels of gratitude that may be associated with such stressful life events. This is an issue that should be appropriately considered by institutional managers when selecting, training, and supporting staff chosen to be available to undertake this kind of work.

One of the first issues to be addressed by responding agencies is the development of selection criteria to be used in assembling those individuals who will be called upon to respond to such MFI especially where identification is the major component. This may include the development of an appropriate training program and such training should include prominent awareness of the potential risk faced by operatives involved in these incidents and also advice on the interventions that may be available or protective factors that should be considered (Mahaffey et al., 2021).

In addressing the adverse effects of these incidents, the need for pre-event interventions should be emphasized. For example, educational information about the effects of particular types of events such as terrorist attacks, natural catastrophes or biological threats and of the potential consequences of exposure to such events may assist forensic workers to address the MFI and devise strategies to prevent or minimize adverse impacts. Additionally, it is important to understand the ways in which factors associated with the event such as number of fatalities, condition of the remains, rate of recovery, and availability of a manifest may influence the duration of the identification process. It must be recognized that factors which lengthen the identification process will likely influence the duration of stress exposure for the employees (Brondolo, 2004). Exercises that simulate disasters allow responders and forensic investigators to plan and practice effective responses to such incidents and in this way, the preparation may reduce the degree to which these events and their sequelae are perceived as threatening. Additionally, workers may improve skills and gain in confidence in respect of the equipment required to complete body recovery and identification. This training will also ensure that safety precautions and equipment can be confirmed, thereby improving the confidence and resilience of response workers.

It should be recognized that such disaster exercises and training can also provide the opportunity for the workers to recognize the concept of and potential for stress and stress responses and to learn to anticipate their own emotional responses in such situations. In such guided exercises, individuals can learn to recognize their own emotional reactions during such a drill. In addition, their concerns about other stressful situations can be anticipated so that appropriate responses can be designed and implemented. Especially in that part of the identification process whereby antemortem information is collected from victims' families, such preparatory and training exercises can provide guidance for forensic workers who are likely to interact with those families. Indeed, it may be appropriate to provide opportunities for training MFI responders to interact with family members who have already experienced disasters as the responders can then identify and learn to cope with their own reactions to the victims' families' needs.

Although the responding agency may not be able to control the size or nature of the disaster or the specific type of response required, it is appropriate that the agency should attempt to manage the mental and physical responses of its responders to that incident. Some aspects of the incident will be beyond the control of the agency, but it is incumbent on managers to ensure that all individuals involved in the MFI response are provided with maximum facilities and resources whether physical, psychological, or emotional to minimize any post-event adverse effects. As managers prepare disaster plans including the development of emergency training drills, they should identify potential stress-inducing situations. As mentioned above, these stresses can include the intense time pressure imposed by the public or by political masters demanding rapid identification of victims. Additionally, operators will be confronted with individuals facing serious outcomes as a result of the MFI, such as potential loss of loved ones and homes. These intense demands can be quite threatening, and it is important to ensure that MFI responders are supported and reassured that the many demands created by the MFI are shared widely and that an extensive range of resources should be available. The agency managing the response must also ensure that their organizational structure and staffing hours are flexible and appropriate for the personnel available, and the response required by the particular incident.

The support provided to MFI responders is obviously the principal responsibility of the responding agency although in real terms, the importance of group response cannot be undervalued, and the group interaction of responders should be maximized and encouraged throughout the whole incident. This may be treated as a formal exercise in which there is group discussion, sometimes referred to as debriefing, or it may be treated as a more informal relaxed process where the group members relax and interact with one another often in an environment totally unrelated to the confronting situation in which the identification process has to be conducted. So informal timeout or relaxation can be very beneficial although it must be regarded that this needs to be managed and controlled by the agency to ensure that it is properly focused and that all potentially affected workers are covered by this process. It should be noted that the concept of debriefing is not universally accepted as it is occasionally associated with an increased focus on the disaster with the potential for actually increasing the adverse psychological response of participants (Wagner, 2005). This group interaction is sometimes referred to as the buddy/support system and is a very important part of the management of the psychological care of MFI responders (Raphael et al., 1995; Raphael & Wooding, 2004).

Ultimately, support services after the incident are of great importance in managing ongoing psychological stresses and minimizing subsequent adverse effects. It is generally accepted by disaster response managers that appropriate access to counselling should be made available to all responders although it is necessary to ensure that this is handled in a sensitive and confidential manner (Brooks et al., 2020). The responses of operatives and their reactions to different disasters vary dramatically, especially in respect of the different family, social, and psychological arrangements faced by all the different individuals. Some operators will seek outside intervention whereas others would prefer for it to be regarded as personal and confidential and it is necessary for the managing agency to recognize this extensive range of personal, psychological, and social needs among all the individuals. Included in this post-operational response should be a mechanism whereby reintegration in the individual's normal work and social environment can be facilitated and supported. This is especially an issue where the individual operative has been seconded from an agency not normally involved in such disaster response but who must return to his/her agency after the work conducted in the mass fatality location is finalized. This assistance may include coordination of support services from the original employing agency and ensuring that the MFI responding agency provides the original employing unit with appropriate information and supportive advice.

Finally, it is appropriate to discuss how the recommended support arrangements outlined above would be applied in the situation of John, the recently bereaved response officer from the vignette. In such an incident, early responders would include emergency workers who would have little exposure to mass fatality and the managing agency would of necessity be required to note that the exposure to such bodily disruption could be very distressing. Ongoing support, both personal and institutional, would be necessary for all the workers exposed to the injured, deceased, and fragmented human remains and involved in the recovery and identification of those remains. It would be necessary for agency managers to recognize that responders would be exposed to deceased children and that this could be a source of significant stress to many of the operatives. It would be appropriate for support to be provided for the group and also for individuals in that environment. In particular, it would be advised that all responding officers are at least provided with the option of independent and personal support. Because of his recent bereavement, John will need close monitoring and assistance and this support may be required for years after the event.

References

Brondolo, E., Wellington, R., Brady, N., Libby, D., & Brondolo, T.J. (2008). Mechanism and strategies for preventing post-traumatic stress disorder in forensic workers responding to mass fatality incidents. *Journal of Forensic and Legal Medicine*, *15*, 78–88. doi:10.1016/j.jflm.2007.04.007

Brondolo, E., Wellington, R., Brondolo, T. J., & Delahanty, D. (2012). Work-related predictors of psychological distress among medical examiner and coroner personnel. *Academic Forensic Pathology*, *2*, 80–91. doi:10.23907/2012.011

Brondolo, T. J. (2004). Resource requirements for medical examiner response to mass fatality incidents. *Medico-Legal Journal of Ireland*, *10*, 91–102

Brooks, S., Amlot, R., Rubin, G.J., & Greenberg, N. (2020). Psychological resilience and post-traumatic growth in disaster-exposed organisations: overview of the literature. *BMJ Military Health*, *166*, 52–56. doi:10.1136/jramc-2017-000876

Brooks, S. K., Dunn, R., Sage, C. A., Amlôt, R., Greenberg, N., & Rubin, G. J. (2015). Risk and resilience factors affecting the psychological wellbeing of individuals deployed in humanitarian relief roles after a disaster. *Journal of Mental Health*, *24*, 385–413. doi:10.3109/09638237.2015.1057334

Cordner, S., & Ellingham, S. T. (2017). Two halves make a whole: both first responders and experts are needed for the management and identification of the dead in large disasters. *Forensic Science International*, *279*, 60–64. doi:10.1016/j.forsciint.2017.07.020

Garbern, S. C., Ebbeling, L. G., & Bartels, S. A. (2016). A systematic review of health outcomes among disaster and humanitarian responders. *Prehospital and Disaster Medicine*, *31*, 635–642. doi:10.1017/S1049023X16000832

Glaysher, E., Vallis, J., & Reeves, P. (2016). Post traumatic stress disorder and the forensic radiographer. *Radiography*, *22*, e212–e215. doi:10.1016/j.radi.2016.04.010

Interpol (2018). Interpol Disaster Victim Identification Guide. Retrieved 16 September 2022 from https://www.interpol.int/How-we-work/Forensics/Disaster-Victim-Identification-DVI

Leppma, M., Mnatsakanova, A., Sarkisian, K., Scott, O., Adjeroh, L., Andrew, M. E.,Violant, J. M., & McCanlies, E. C. (2018). Stressful life events and posttraumatic growth among police officers: A cross-sectional study. *Stress and Health, 34,* 175–186. doi:10.1002/smi.2772

Levin, A. P., Putney, H., Crimmins, D., & McGrath, J. G. (2021). Secondary traumatic stress, burnout, compassion satisfaction, and perceived organizational trauma readiness in forensic science professionals. *Journal of Forensic Sciences, 66,* 1758–1769. doi:10.1111/1556-4029.14747

Mahaffey, B. L., Mackin, D. M., Rosen, J., Schwartz, R. M., Taioli, E., & Gonzalez, A. (2021). The disaster worker resiliency training program: a randomized clinical trial. *International Archives of Occupational and Environmental Health, 94,* 9–21. doi:10.1007/s00420-020-01552-3

Nagamine, M., Harada, N., Shigemura, J., Dobashi, K., Yoshiga, M., Esaki, N., Tanaka, M., Tanichi, M., Yoshino, A., & Shimizu, K. (2016). The effects of living environment on disaster workers: a one–year longitudinal study. *BMC Psychiatry, 16,* 1–7. doi:10.1186/s12888-016-1058-4

Quevillon, R. P., Gray, B. L., Erickson, S. E., Gonzalez, E. D., & Jacobs, G. A. (2016). Helping the helpers: assisting staff and volunteer workers before, during, and after disaster relief operations. *Journal of Clinical Psychology, 72,* 1348–1363. doi:10.1002/jclp.22336

Raphael, B., Meldrum, L., & McFarlane, A. C. (1995). Does debriefing after psychological trauma work? *BMJ, 310*(6993), 1479–1480. doi:10.1136/bmj.310.6993.1479

Raphael, B., & Wooding, S. (2004). Debriefing: Its evolution and current status. *Psychiatric Clinics, 27,* 407–423. doi:10.1016/j.psc.2004.03.003

Sakuma, A., Takahashi, Y., Ueda, I., Sato, H., Katsura, M., Abe, M., Nagao, A., Suzuki, Y., Kakizaki, M., Tsuji, I., Matsuoka, H., & Matsumoto, K. (2015). Post-traumatic stress disorder and depression prevalence and associated risk factors among local disaster relief and reconstruction workers fourteen months after the Great East Japan Earthquake: a cross-sectional study. *BMC Psychiatry, 15,* 1–13. doi:10.1186/s12888-015-0440-y

Tedeschi, R. G., Shakespeare-Finch, J., Taku, K., & Calhoun, L. G. (2018). *Posttraumatic Growth: Theory, Research and Applications.* New York: Routledge

Wagner, S. L. (2005). Emergency response service personnel and the critical incident stress debriefing debate. *International Journal of Emergency Mental Health, 7,* 33–41

Humanitarian Workers

15

Gülşah Kurt, Mohamed Elshazly,
Olga Rebolledo, Ruth Wells, and
Simon Rosenbaum

Mary and Aisha

Mary is a female psychologist working at an international non-governmental organization providing health services to the internally displaced Syrian community inside Syria. Since the conflict began in 2011, millions of people have been forced to leave their homes. Almost 2 million Syrians live in camps in Northwest Syria. As a conflict-affected country, Syria's health infrastructure and facilities were irreversibly destroyed. Only a small number of organizations operating in the area provide humanitarian support. Mary's organization is one of those few to provide psychosocial support services. She was deployed to Syria three years ago after completing an assignment in the Gaza district of Palestine. She provides psychological counseling and therapy to adults and children. Due to the limited provision of mental health services, the number of service users exceeds the capacity of the available staff at her organization. It is not possible for her organization to recruit more staff as the funded projects are coming to an end. Thus, she is forced to see more than ten clients per day, work six days per week, and also provide supervision to her team. Due to the budget shortage, her payment was recently cut off. Mary feels exhausted and lacks the energy to get up in the morning. She constantly questions herself and if her effort is worth the trouble that she has been through, separation from her family and friends, earning a low wage, and constant stress. She does not see a point in helping people anymore. She is embarrassed to think that those people are not trying hard enough to adapt to the situation and always want others to help them. Two days ago, Mary became emotionally overwhelmed at work and fought with one of her colleagues, Aisha.

Aisha is a Syrian female social worker. She had to leave her home in the capital and move to Idlib, where the organization is based. She lost her husband and children two years ago due to the bombing in her hometown. She now lives with her mother. Aisha thinks that it is her duty and responsibility to help her community. Although she

DOI: 10.4324/9781003292807-17

finds her job inherently satisfying, she is having difficulty working with children and female clients who also lost their families. She feels agitated and anxious after her sessions with these clients. She often cries and feels extreme fear that she will never have a normal life and that she will also lose her mother. She sees her husband and children happy together as a family in her dreams and has visions of them dying in front of her eyes. She sleeps no more than three hours per day and always feels exhausted. She is also tired of unequal treatment of Syrian and international staff at her organization and had a recent fight with Mary.

Globally, natural disasters, conflict, violence, and economic and political turmoil pose a significant threat to the health, security, and well-being of communities. Humanitarian emergencies occur when crisis situations exceed the capacity and resources of local communities to fight back against the negative consequences (Inter-Agency Standing Committee [IASC], 2007). Humanitarian workers come from diverse professional backgrounds (e.g., healthcare staff, case managers, administrative staff, and disaster relief workers) and provide a wide range of aid and assistance (e.g., protection of civilians, supplying basic materials and healthcare) during and/or in the aftermath of crisis in emergency settings (Stoddard et al., 2019). Characterized by uncertainty, insecurity, and safety concerns, working in humanitarian emergencies is inherently traumatizing (IASC, 2007). The Aid Worker Security Report (Stoddard et al., 2022) revealed that humanitarian workers often encounter traumatic events, such as airstrikes/shelling, kidnaps, injuries, and physical and sexual assaults. Although the number of major attacks has decreased since 2019, more humanitarian workers have died, mainly due to shootings and airstrikes/shelling in 2022. Over the past few decades, the ongoing conflict has made South Sudan, Afghanistan, and Syria the most dangerous and fragile emergency contexts for humanitarian workers (Stoddard et al., 2019). In addition to perils and risks in emergencies, adverse working conditions including long hours, low wages, and limited support are notoriously challenging (Brooks et al., 2016). Given potentially traumatic events (PTEs) and work-related stressors, humanitarian workers are at risk of experiencing mental health problems including depression, anxiety, posttraumatic stress disorder (PTSD), and burnout (Brooks et al., 2016; Jachens et al., 2019; Strohmeier & Scholte, 2015). In this chapter, we provide an overview of extant studies on the prevalence of and associated factors for mental health problems among HWs. Then, we discuss the occurrence of posttraumatic growth among HWs despite the challenging nature of humanitarian work. Lastly, we discuss emerging prevention and treatment-focused programs promoting positive mental health and wellbeing among HWs.

Mental Health Problems among Humanitarian Workers

Estimated prevalence rates of poor mental health in HWs are comparable to crisis-affected populations (Connorton et al., 2012; Lopes Cardozo et al., 2013; Putnam et al., 2009). In a study of national HWs in Sri Lanka, Lopes Cardozo et al. (2013) found the estimated prevalence of PTSD, depression, and anxiety was 19%, 58%, and 53%, respectively. Similarly, one in five HWs providing services to Iraqi refugees in Jordan was at risk of developing PTSD. Almost half were likely to suffer from depression and anxiety (Eriksson et al., 2013). In their study with national HWs in Northern Uganda, Ager and colleagues (2012) reported slightly higher rates of PTSD (26%), depression (68%), and anxiety (53%). In a more recent study with national and international HWs in South Sudan, estimated prevalence rates were reported as 24% for PTSD, 39% for depression, and 38% for anxiety (Strohmeier et al., 2018). Further, 10 to 30% of HWs are likely to develop hazardous drinking and alcohol use problems (De Jong et al., 2021; Strohmeier et al., 2018). Suicidal ideation can increase almost three-fold after an assignment (Wang et al., 2016). A systematic review of trauma-related mental health problems among national HWs showed that the prevalence rates widely varied between 6% and 42% for PTSD, 4% and 68% for depression, and 8% and 58% for anxiety, depending on the study and sample characteristics including assessment methods and the context (Strohmeier & Scholte, 2015). Discrepancies in the prevalence of mental health problems across studies are best evident in the recent study conducted by De Jong et al. (2021). In this study conducted with international HWs, they found that self-administered measurements led to overinflated estimates compared to clinical interviews. The latter found the estimates of PTSD, depression, and anxiety as 0.3%, 1.3%, and 6.6%, respectively, while these rates were reported three times higher for anxiety (20%), eight times higher for PTSD (2.4%), and 25 times higher for depression (32.4%) when assessed by self-report instruments. Therefore, findings related to the prevalence of mental health problems should be interpreted with caution.

The International Classification of Disease (11th edition) (ICD-11) (World Health Organization; WHO, 2019) defines burnout as "a syndrome that results from chronic workplace stress that has not been successfully managed." Cumulative evidence shows that burnout is highly prevalent among professionals like healthcare workers (Rotenstein et al., 2018; Woo et al., 2020), mental health professionals (O'Connor et al., 2018), police officers (García-Rivera et al., 2020), and teachers (García-Carmona et al., 2019). Although burnout is not conceived as a mental health condition, it is associated with far-reaching physical and mental health outcomes such as depression, anxiety, physical pain, and even mortality (Salvagioni et al., 2017). HWs are also at risk of burnout given the excessive emotional, physical, and interpersonal involvement in their work. Burnout needs to be understood as a complexity of factors associated with humanitarian assistance, such as the dynamics of relationships established with direct supervisors, the volatile and unstable security situation, restrictions on mobility, and the lifestyle that does not allow people to establish roots in one place that can be called "home." In a large cross-sectional survey study of international and national HWs working in more than 100 emergencies, 10% to 40% of HWs reported elevated symptoms of burnout, with 32% for emotional exhaustion (EE), 43% for personal accomplishment (PA), and 10% for depersonalization (DP) (Jachens et al., 2019). Previous findings also support these results among national HWs in Uganda (25–50%) (Ager et al., 2012) and a mixed group of HWs in South Sudan (19–24%) (Strohmeier et al., 2018). In a longitudinal study, international HWs showed higher symptoms of EE and DP at post-deployment than at pre-deployment. Symptoms of burnout remained high at the 3–6 month follow-up assessment (Lopes Cardozo et al., 2012). HWs are most likely to suffer from the emotional exhaustion component of burnout, with the rates ranging from 24% to 50%. This is evidence of the emotionally taxing nature of humanitarian work, making HWs susceptible to mental health problems. HWs' deteriorated mental health can lead to adverse organizational outcomes including staff turnover, loss of institutional knowledge and productivity, financial costs, and reduced quality of care (Welton-Mitchell, 2023). Therefore, it is necessary to understand the risk and protective factors to promote HWs' mental health and wellbeing and prevent adverse outcomes. In the following section, we provide an overview of the risk and protective factors for mental health considering three categories: 1) emergency-related factors; 2) work-related factors; and 3) personal and/or professional factors (Table 1).

Emergency-related Factors

Humanitarian emergencies are volatile, insecure, and perilous settings that expose HWs to potentially traumatic events (PTEs). HWs are likely to have minimal or no access to basic services such as food, water, sanitation, shelter, and safety equipment (Brooks et al., 2015). Due to security concerns, they may not be allowed to move or travel as much as they want during the assignment (De Jong et al., 2021, Strohmeimer et al., 2018). Natural conditions (e.g., excessive heat, cold, noise) might further exacerbate the working conditions of HWs as most emergencies occur in geographically challenging areas. These create a sense of personal threat and danger and increase vulnerability to mental health problems (Brooks et al., 2016).

Almost all HWs are directly or indirectly exposed to various traumatic events. The most common first-hand traumatic experiences are exposure to war or combat, physical or sexual assault, injuries, and kidnappings (De Jong et al., 2021; Stoddard et al., 2022). The number of PTEs experienced is associated with increased risk for depression, anxiety, PTSD, and burnout (De Jong et al., 2021; Lopes Cardozo et al., 2012). Further, secondary exposure to traumatic events is ubiquitous as the job of HWs entails frequent interaction with potentially traumatized individuals. Previous findings show that HWs are likely to be traumatized by listening to the experiences of those who provide aid (Eriksson et al., 2013; Lopes Cardozo et al., 2013). Secondary traumatization elevates the risk of experiencing physical and mental health problems such as PTSD among HWs (Lopes Cardozo et al., 2013; Rizkalla & Siegel, 2019).

Work-related Factors

Work-related factors, including organizational factors and working conditions, are the key determinants of the day-to-day experiences of HWs. Although the emergency setting factors are of critical importance for mental health, work-related factors can be more predictive of mental health outcomes as those are more proximal and pervasive in HWs' day-to-day operations (Ager et al., 2012; Connorton et al., 2012; Lopes Cardozo et al., 2013; Strohmeier et al., 2018). In this section, we provide an overview of organizational factors and working conditions that promote or impair the mental health of HWs.

The type of organizations that HWs work at was found to be an important factor for mental health. A systematic review showed that working at the United Nations (UN) and related agencies were associated with better mental health outcomes than at national or international organizations (Strohmeier & Scholte, 2015). This is attributed to the formal structure and policies of UN agencies to provide staff support and protect HWs' mental health. Interagency communication in the same emergency setting can facilitate the aid work and reduce psychological distress as it helps coordination of distribution of services and reduces the tension and rivalry among HWs, especially among national and international HWs (Brooks et al., 2015). Another organizational factor is perceived organizational support during and in the aftermath of the assignment. This refers to both emotional and professional support, including support from managers/supervisors and colleagues, availability of support services, benefits, and training. In a systematic review, Brooks et al. (2016) reported that a supportive work environment and supervisor support reduced the risk of mental health problems and turnover intention and promoted job satisfaction and engagement. Further, higher team cohesion and availability of supportive measures were associated with lower burnout and psychological distress among national HWs in Uganda (Ager et al., 2012). Aldamman et al. (2019) showed that perceived organizational support might reduce the feeling of helplessness and increase the perceived self-efficacy among HWs, promoting their wellbeing. On the other hand, lack of communication with and clear direction from managers and conflict between colleagues can adversely impact HWs' mental health (Brooks et al., 2016; Young et al., 2018).

Working conditions such as long hours without adequate breaks and low wages can be challenging for HWs. Lack of recognition for their effort and experiencing or witnessing differential treatment between colleagues might add to the existing difficulties and increase the risk of experiencing mental health difficulties (Brooks et al., 2016; De Jong et al., 2021; Young & Pakenham, 2021). These stressors can create the perception of imbalance between the effort that HWs exert on their work and the rewards they receive in turn. Higher perceived effort-reward imbalance might lead to burnout, especially emotional exhaustion among HWs (Aldamman et al., 2019).

During their work, HWs face morally challenging situations where they need to make difficult decisions and choices. Such challenging situations involve deciding whom to prioritize in providing aid, being forced to provide lower-quality care, acting outside of the competence area, overlooking potentially risky situations, and more (Gustavsson et al., 2020). Moral injury can occur if HWs must act or witness behaviors that transgress their moral values and beliefs. Moral injury is usually accompanied by strong emotions such as guilt, anger, helplessness, and frustration, which might precipitate or exacerbate mental health problems (Williamson et al., 2018). However, support from organizations and colleagues might mitigate the risk of mental health problems (Gustavsson et al., 2022).

Despite challenging working conditions, HWs are likely to find their work with affected individuals meaningful and pleasant (Eriksson et al., 2013; Gustavsson et al., 2020). Strohmeier et al. (2018) found that working directly with service users might reduce the risk of emotional exhaustion as it is likely to be satisfying. However, it is important to note that too much emotional involvement and identification with the service users can lead to secondary traumatization and thereby increase the risk for PTSD (Brooks et al., 2016). Overcommitment to their work with the service users might also deplete the emotional capacity and resources of HWs and lead to emotional exhaustion (Jachens et al., 2019).

Personal and Professional Factors

National HWs are at higher risk of experiencing mental health problems than their international counterparts (Eriksson et al., 2013; Lopes Cardozo et al., 2013; Strohmeier et al., 2018). Coming from the crisis-affected community, national HWs must contend with the stress related to providing services to their community while dealing with work-related stressors simultaneously. They also experience more traumatic events than international HWs (Stoddard et al., 2022). National HWs are more likely to experience unfair workplace treatment such as lower wages and fewer

Table 15.1 Summary of risk and protective factors across three categories

	Risk factors	Protective factors
Emergency-related factors	Challenging natural conditions (e.g., excessive heat, cold, or noise)	Sense of safety and security
	Lack of access to basic equipment and service (e.g., access to clean water, sanitation, and shelter)	
	Direct exposure to traumatic events (e.g., physical and/or sexual violence, injuries, kidnaps, etc.)	
	Indirect exposure to traumatic events via work with the affected communities	
Work-related factors	Long working hours without adequate breaks	Working at the UN and related agencies
	Low wages	Interagency communication in the emergency setting
	Lack of recognition and appreciation	Perceived organizational support during and aftermath of the assignment (support from managers/ supervisors and colleagues, availability of support services, etc.)
	Differential treatment among workers	Finding meaning in the humanitarian work
	Perceived effort-reward imbalance	
	Facing morally challenging situations	
	Overcommitment to work	
Personal & Professional Factors	National background	Older age
	Female gender	Positive cognitive reappraisal strategies

Table 15.1 (Continued)

	Risk factors	Protective factors
	Volunteers	Religiosity and spirituality
	Previous history of trauma and psychiatric disorders	
	Using dysfunctional coping strategies (e.g., avoidance, denial, self-distancing, and behavioral disengagement)	

career opportunities than international HWs (Ager et al., 2012). Further, volunteering in humanitarian work puts one at elevated risk of experiencing mental health problems (Young & Pakenham, 2021). Professionals are likely to receive psychological training that prepare them for the potential challenges in the field (Young & Pakenham, 2021). However, the provision of training and preparedness for volunteers is minimal (Brooks et al., 2016).

Older age is a protective factor against higher level of psychological distress and burnout (Eriksson et al., 2013; Jachens et al., 2019; Young & Pakenham, 2021). Female gender appears to be an important risk factor for mental health (Strohmeier & Scholte, 2015). In their study with international HWs, De Jong et al. (2021) showed that female and male HWs experienced similar level of work-related stressors, but females were disproportionately exposed to sexual violence and assault. They encountered more problems related to organizational support and team communication, and they felt more powerless and helpless. Gender-based and sexual violence and lack of support might increase the risk for mental health problems among females. Previous history of trauma and psychiatric disorders are also found to be risk factors for increasing HWs' vulnerability to humanitarian work-related stressors (Brooks et al., 2016).

The way individuals cope with the stressors determines the psychological aftermath of the stressful event (Lazarus & Folkman, 1984). Studies among both national and international HWs indicated the positive association between dysfunctional coping and mental health problems such as depression and anxiety. Using dysfunctional coping strategies such as avoidance, denial, self-distancing, and behavioral disengagement is harmful for mental health (Lopes Cardozo et al., 2013; Strohmeier et al., 2018). On the other hand, religiosity and spirituality act as a buffer against psychological distress related to humanitarian work (Young & Pakenham, 2021). Positive cognitive reappraisal strategies such as acceptance of uncontrollable aspects of the work and focusing on the importance of the work can promote well-being (Young et al., 2018).

Posttraumatic Growth among HWs

Despite demanding working conditions and potentially traumatic events, the majority of HWs can maintain functioning and show positive psychological outcomes. The concept of posttraumatic growth (PTG) can help understand the positive changes among HWs. A growing number of studies also support the occurrence of PTG among HWs. Veronese et al. (2017) showed that experiencing potentially traumatic events during an assignment was associated with higher level of psychological distress and negative affect as well as PTG among humanitarian healthcare professionals in Palestine. PTG can also mitigate the negative impacts of traumatic experiences on wellbeing by enabling HWs to reevaluate their experiences in a positive way. Further, in a study with HWs working at Red Cross Organization in China, Wen et al. (2021) found that PTG and PTSD can co-occur in response to stressful experiences in the field. Presence of PTG does not refute the fact that HWs are likely to show heightened levels of mental health problems during or after their assignment. Experiencing initial psychological distress is a prerequisite to develop PTG (Tedeschi & Calhoun, 2004). Yet, deliberate positive thinking and reconstructing traumatic experiences might foster psychological growth in the face of adversities that HWS experience in their work. Mindfulness can help HWs to develop PTG as it is related to one's ability to accept things without judgment and stay in the present moment (Wen et al., 2021). In a four-year follow up study with disaster relief workers, Nishi et al. (2016) reported that PTG is likely to occur even several years after a deployment and is associated with positive work outcomes such as higher work engagement.

Meaning of the work and feelings of being useful are of critical importance to understand positive outcomes as HWs are motivated by altruistic aims and the meaning of humanitarian work (Young et al., 2018). Finding meaning in their work and ability to make meaningful contributions can protect HWs against adverse psychological outcomes and foster psychological flexibility to continue their work aligned with their altruistic values (Young et al., 2022). Further, HWs are likely to see their stressful experiences as opportunities to learn and grow. Such experiences are considered an inseparable part of their work. Managing morally distressing situations promotes personal and professional growth among HWs and self-confidence in their abilities. HWs can feel motivated to engage in creative and constructive ways to solve problems in the future (Gustavsson et al., 2022).

Supporting the Mental Health of Humanitarian Workers

In the opening vignette, we described the difficulties experienced by Mary and Aisha, two humanitarian workers providing support at the same organization. Although they reported different types of stressors, both seem to suffer from mental health problems. What actions are needed to alleviate their suffering and promote well-being? Existing studies extensively focused on understanding mental health problems and associated factors. Therefore, less is known as to how to effectively address mental health problems and support the well-being of HWs. In this section, we provide an overview of available evidence-based interventions and strategies to protect and promote HWs' mental health.

Strohmeier and colleagues (2019) conducted a study with 210 HWs in South Sudan to identify the priority areas and effective strategies to promote mental health. Organizational policies ensuring safety and security of staff were identified as the main condition for protecting mental health. Effective risk management protocols and strategies should be formed and implemented to mitigate safety concerns among HWs. Additionally, living conditions of those in the field should be improved by meeting the basic needs such as proper shelter, food, access to clean water, and internet (Brooks et al., 2016). As working conditions are primary determinants of the mental health of HWs, it is important to create an equal, fair, and ethical work environment. This can be achieved by reducing workload and working hours, providing career opportunities, good compensation, and equal treatment among staff (Strohmeier et al., 2019).

Supportive organizational policies such as availability of support services, benefits, and training are conducive to mental health (Brooks et al., 2016). Availability of psychosocial support does not guarantee its utilization among HWs. Professional help-seeking is minimal among HWs. De Jong et al. (2021) found that less than ten percent of international HWs utilized mental health services after their assignments. Similarly, only 11% of national HWs reported that they were currently using mental health services while 25% had ever sought psychosocial help. Cockcroft-McKay and Eiroa-Orosa (2021) identified the barriers for help-seeking among HWs. First, awareness of mental health issues and available services is low among HWs. Many tend to minimize their problems and consider seeking help as a sign of weakness. Considering the excruciating difficulties that individuals they provide care for must endure, HWs might feel guilty complaining. Further, support from organizations and managers plays an important role in determining HWs' help-seeking behavior. Otherwise, lack of such support might stigmatize seeking professional help among HWs and fuel anxiety and worry about their career and relationships at work. Therefore, to promote mental health, it is necessary to identify the barriers at different levels – personal, organizational, and contextual – and target those amenable to change.

Among supportive organizational policies, providing pre-deployment training can shield HWs against adverse mental health outcomes by equipping them with necessary skills and knowledge. In a systematic review, Brooks et al. (2018) showed pre-disaster trainings can increase self-confidence and knowledge of HWs assigned to disaster relief work.

These trainings include psychoeducation about common stressors and mental health problems among HWs, effective stress coping strategies, and resources for further help. HWs generally find preparedness trainings helpful to prepare them for an assignment and reduce interpersonal difficulties. Such trainings can also increase awareness and familiarity related to mental health problems and thereby facilitate help-seeking among HWs.

Psychosocial support provided after an assignment has also been found to be effective in reducing psychological distress. de Fouchier & Kedia (2018) tested the effectiveness of a group-based single session stress management intervention on the mental health of national aid workers in Central Africa. The intervention included two main components: psychoeducation on common traumatic reactions and effective coping strategies. After the intervention, participants showed significant reduction in their symptoms of depression, anxiety, and PTSD. In another study, a meditation-based intervention was associated with significant improvement in psychological distress and increased capacity for effective stress coping (Waelde et al., 2008). Further, psychological debriefing is one of the most widely used interventions for potentially traumatized HWs. Psychological debriefing aims to help individuals to process traumatic experiences and emotions to reduce risk for mental health problems. It includes deliberate discussion of traumatic experiences and associated feelings. Previous studies on psychological debriefing showed mixed findings (Rose et al., 2002). Brooks et al. (2018) showed that debriefing might even be harmful as it is likely to trigger traumatic memories and result in re-traumatization if provided on one occasion. Despite its wide use, psychological debriefing is not recommended for recently traumatized individuals to reduce the risk of PTSD and related conditions (World Health Organization, 2012). Psychological first aid (PFA) has yielded promising results so far as a safe and scalable alternative to debriefing. A review by Corey et al. (2021) showed that PFA could reduce emotional distress and increase adaptive capacity by providing a safe, supportive, and practical space to share traumatic experiences and normalize stress reactions among HWs. When provided in a group format, it can help build peer support networks and enhance a sense of connectedness. It can also reduce stigma and reluctance related to help-seeking by increasing knowledge and awareness of mental health. As PFA can be provided before, during, and after an assignment, it can serve as both a preventive and treatment option to promote mental health.

To effectively address mental health issues among HWs, strategies or program targeting factors at multiple levels are needed. The multi-layered six-month support program implemented by Othman et al. (2018) exemplifies the importance of a multi-component need-based support program to enhance work outcomes among HWs. In this study, they first identified the needs and challenges of healthcare workers in a conflict-affected area of Syria. Healthcare workers identified several challenges at contextual, individual, relationship, and management levels. Based on these challenges and needs, the research team iteratively designed the content and structure of the support program with the healthcare workers. The final program included strategies to promote individual well-being, enhance skills, build team cohesion, and establish policies and guidelines for self-care in the organization. The program resulted in improved work outcomes for healthcare workers such as reduction in role ambiguity and improvements in relationships at work and working conditions.

There is a growing interest in identifying effective strategies to protect HWs against adverse mental health and work outcomes. Yet, the literature on evidence-based interventions and programs is at a nascent stage. Existing findings have yet to elucidate what works for whom and why. Some groups of HWs, such as national HWs, females, and volunteers, are at particular risk of experiencing mental health difficulties. Identification of those at risk is important to provide timely support. Comprehensive, needs-based, multi-layered support programs are warranted to address mental health needs of HWs and promote positive psychological changes.

Conclusion

Humanitarian workers are at increased risk of experiencing mental health problems. Mary and Aisha portray mental health difficulties experienced by international and national HWs. This chapter reviewed the prevalence of common mental health difficulties among humanitarian workers and presented the risk and protective factors under three categories: 1) emergency-related factors; 2) work-related factors; and 3) personal and professional factors. Given that humanitarian workers are likely to maintain functioning and even show positive psychological outcomes, this chapter portrayed supporting evidence for posttraumatic growth among humanitarian workers. Lastly, we reviewed the available evidence-based strategies and interventions at multiple levels to address mental health needs and promote the wellbeing of HWs. Future studies are warranted to focus on positive aspects of humanitarian work and uncover potential avenues to promote the mental health and wellbeing of HWs.

References

Ager, A., Pasha, E., Yu, G., Duke, T., Eriksson, C., & Cardozo, B. L. (2012). Stress, Mental Health, and Burnout in National Humanitarian Aid Workers in Gulu, Northern Uganda: Stress in National Humanitarian Workers in Uganda. *Journal of Traumatic Stress, 25,* 713–720. doi:10.1002/jts.21764

Aldamman, K., Tamrakar, T., Dinesen, C., Wiedemann, N., Murphy, J., Hansen, M., Elsiddig Badr, E., Reid, T., & Vallières, F. (2019). Caring for the mental health of humanitarian volunteers in traumatic contexts: The importance of organisational support. *European Journal of Psychotraumatology, 10*, 1694811. doi:10.1080/20008198.2019.1694811

Brooks, S. K., Dunn, R., Sage, C. A. M., Amlôt, R., Greenberg, N., & Rubin, G. J. (2015). Risk and resilience factors affecting the psychological wellbeing of individuals deployed in humanitarian relief roles after a disaster. *Journal of Mental Health, 24*, 385–413. doi:10.3109/09638237.2015.1057334

Brooks, S. K., Dunn, R., Amlôt, R., Greenberg, N., & Rubin, G. J. (2016). Social and occupational factors associated with psychological distress and disorder among disaster responders: A systematic review. *BMC Psychology, 4*, 18. doi:10.1186/s40359-016-0120-9

Brooks, S. K., Dunn, R., Amlôt, R., Greenberg, N., & Rubin, G. J. (2018). Training and post-disaster interventions for the psychological impacts on disaster-exposed employees: A systematic review. *Journal of Mental Health, 15*, 1–25. doi:10.1080/09638237.2018.1437610

Cockcroft-McKay, C., & Eiroa-Orosa, F. J. (2021). Barriers to accessing psychosocial support for humanitarian aid workers: A mixed methods inquiry. *Disasters, 45*, 762–796. https://onlinelibrary.wiley.com/doi/full/10.1111/disa.12449

Connorton, E., Perry, M. J., Hemenway, D., & Miller, M. (2012). Humanitarian Relief Workers and Trauma-related Mental Illness. *Epidemiologic Reviews, 34*, 145–155. doi:10.1093/epirev/mxr026

Corey, J., Vallières, F., Frawley, T., De Brún, A., Davidson, S., & Gilmore, B. (2021). A Rapid Realist Review of Group Psychological First Aid for Humanitarian Workers and Volunteers. *International Journal of Environmental Research and Public Health, 18*, 1452. doi:10.3390/ijerph18041452

de Fouchier, C., & Kedia, M. (2018). Trauma-related mental health problems and effectiveness of a stress management group in national humanitarian workers in the Central African Republic. *Intervention, 16*, 103. doi:10.4103/INTV.INTV_9_18

De Jong, K., Martinmäki, S. E., Te Brake, H., Haagen, J. F. G., & Kleber, R. J. (2021). Mental and physical health of international humanitarian aid workers on short-term assignments: Findings from a prospective cohort study. *Social Science & Medicine, 285*, 114268. doi:10.1016/j.socscimed.2021.114268

Eriksson, C. B., Lopes Cardozo, B., Ghitis, F., Sabin, M., Gotway Crawford, C., Zhu, J., Rijnen, B., & Kaiser, R. (2013). Factors Associated With Adverse Mental Health Outcomes in Locally Recruited Aid Workers Assisting Iraqi Refugees in Jordan. *Journal of Aggression, Maltreatment & Trauma, 22*, 660–680. doi:10.1080/10926771.2013.803506

García-Carmona, M., Marín, M. D., & Aguayo, R. (2019). Burnout syndrome in secondary school teachers: A systematic review and meta-analysis. *Social Psychology of Education, 22,* 189–208. doi:10.1007/s11218-018-9471-9

García-Rivera, B. R., Olguín-Tiznado, J. E., Aranibar, M. F., Ramírez-Barón, M. C., Camargo-Wilson, C., López-Barreras, J. A., & García-Alcaraz, J. L. (2020). Burnout Syndrome in Police Officers and Its Relationship with Physical and Leisure Activities. *International Journal of Environmental Research and Public Health, 17,* 5586. doi:10.3390/ijerph17155586

Gustavsson, M. E., Arnberg, F. K., Juth, N., & von Schreeb, J. (2020). Moral Distress among Disaster Responders: What is it? *Prehospital and Disaster Medicine, 35,* 212–219. doi:10.1017/S1049023X20000096

Gustavsson, M. E., Juth, N., Arnberg, F. K., & von Schreeb, J. (2022). Dealing with difficult choices: A qualitative study of experiences and consequences of moral challenges among disaster healthcare responders. *Conflict and Health, 16,* 24. doi:10.1186/s13031-022-00456-y

Inter-Agency Standing Committee (2007). IASC guidelines on mental health and psychosocial support in emergency settings. Geneva, Switzerland: IASC 2006. https://interagencystandingcommittee.org/iasc-task-force-mental-health-and-psychosocial-support-emergency-settings/iasc-guidelines-mental-health-and-psychosocial-support-emergency-settings-2007

Jachens, L., Houdmont, J., & Thomas, R. (2019). Effort–reward imbalance and burnout among humanitarian aid workers. *Disasters, 43,* 67–87. doi:10.1111/disa.12288

Lazarus, R. S & Folkman, S. (1984). *The stress concept in the life sciences. Stress, appraisal, and coping.* New York: Springer. https://books.google.com.au/books?hl=en&lr=&id=i-ySQQuUpr8C&oi=fnd&pg=PR5&dq=lazarus+and+folkman+1984&ots=DgKRirgiPc&sig=nJCfERL2AIW7RCOw_NGaVRTG74A#v=onepage&q=lazarus%20and%20folkman%201984&f=false

Lopes Cardozo, B., Gotway Crawford, C., Eriksson, C., Zhu, J., Sabin, M., Ager, A., Foy, D., Snider, L., Scholte, W., Kaiser, R., Olff, M., Rijnen, B., & Simon, W. (2012). Psychological Distress, Depression, Anxiety, and Burnout among International Humanitarian Aid Workers: A Longitudinal Study. *PLoS ONE, 7,* e44948. doi:10.1371/journal.pone.0044948

Lopes Cardozo, B., Sivilli, T. I., Crawford, C., Scholte, W. F., Petit, P., Ghitis, F., Ager, A., & Eriksson, C. (2013). Factors affecting mental health of local staff working in the Vanni region, Sri Lanka. *Psychological Trauma: Theory, Research, Practice, and Policy, 5,* 581–590. doi:10.1037/a0030969

Nishi, D., Kawashima, Y., Noguchi, H., Usuki, M., Yamashita, A., Koido, Y., & Matsuoka, Y. J. (2016). Resilience, post-traumatic growth, and work engagement among health care professionals after the Great East Japan Earthquake: A 4-year prospective follow-up study. *Journal of Occupational Health, 58,* 347–353

O'Connor, K., Muller Neff, D., & Pitman, S. (2018). Burnout in mental health professionals: A systematic review and meta-analysis of prevalence and determinants. *European Psychiatry, 53*, 74–99. doi:10.1016/j.eurpsy.2018.06.003

Othman, M., Steel, Z., Lawsin, C., & Wells, R. (2018). Addressing occupational stress among health staff in non-government controlled Northern Syria: Supporting resilience in a dangerous workplace. *Torture Journal, 28*, 104–123. doi:10.7146/torture.v28i3.111200

Putnam, K. M., Lants, J. I., Townsend, C. L., Gallegos, A. M., Potts, A. A., Roberts, R. C., Cree, E. R., de Villagran, M., Eriksson, D. W., & Foy, D. W. (2009). Exposure to violence, support needs, adjustment, and motivators among Guatemalan humanitarian aid workers. *American Journal of Community Psychology, 44*, 109–115. https://pubmed.ncbi.nlm.nih.gov/19554445/

Rizkalla, N., & Segal, S. P. (2019). Trauma during humanitarian work: the effects on intimacy, wellbeing and PTSD-symptoms. *European Journal of Psychotraumatology, 10*, 1679065.https://www.tandfonline.com/doi/full/10.1080/20008198.2019.1679065

Rose, S. C., Bisson, J., Churchill, R., & Wessely, S. (2002). Psychological debriefing for preventing post traumatic stress disorder (PTSD). *Cochrane Database of Systematic Reviews.* doi:10.1002/14651858.CD000560

Rotenstein, L. S., Torre, M., Ramos, M. A., Rosales, R. C., Guille, C., Sen, S., & Mata, D. A. (2018). Prevalence of Burnout Among Physicians: A Systematic Review. *JAMA, 320*, 1131. doi:10.1001/jama.2018.12777

Salvagioni, D. A. J., Melanda, F. N., Mesas, A. E., González, A. D., Gabani, F. L., & Andrade, S. M. de. (2017). Physical, psychological and occupational consequences of job burnout: A systematic review of prospective studies. *PLOS ONE, 12*, e0185781. doi:10.1371/journal.pone.0185781

Stoddard, A., Harvey, P., Czwarno, M., & Breckenridge, M. (2019). *Aid Worker Security Report Figures at a glance.* https://reliefweb.int/report/world/aid-worker-security-report-figures-glance-2019

Stoddard, A., Harvey, P., Czwarno, M., & Breckenridge, M. (2022). *Aid Worker Security Report 2022 – Collateral violence.* https://www.humanitarianoutcomes.org/AWSR_2022

Strohmeier, H., & Scholte, W. F. (2015). Trauma-related mental health problems among national humanitarian staff: A systematic review of the literature. *European Journal of Psychotraumatology, 6*, 28541. doi:10.3402/ejpt.v6.28541

Strohmeier, H., Scholte, W. F., & Ager, A. (2018). Factors associated with common mental health problems of humanitarian workers in South Sudan. *PLOS ONE, 13*, e0205333. doi:10.1371/journal.pone.0205333

Strohmeier, H., Scholte, W. F., & Ager, A. (2019). How to improve organisational staff support? Suggestions from humanitarian workers in South Sudan. *Intervention, 17*, 40. doi:10.4103/INTV.INTV_22_18

Tedeschi, R. G., & Calhoun, L. G. (2004). TARGET ARTICLE: 'Posttraumatic Growth: Conceptual Foundations and Empirical Evidence'. *Psychological Inquiry, 15,* 1–18. doi:10.1207/s15327965pli1501_01

Veronese, G., Pepe, A., Massaiu, I., De Mol, A.-S., & Robbins, I. (2017). Posttraumatic growth is related to subjective well-being of aid workers exposed to cumulative trauma in Palestine. *Transcultural Psychiatry, 54,* 332–356. doi:10.1177/1363461517706288

Waelde, L. C., Uddo, M., Marquett, R., Ropelato, M., Freightman, S., Pardo, A., & Salazar, J. (2008). A pilot study of meditation for mental health workers following Hurricane Katrina. *Journal of Traumatic Stress, 21,* 497–500. doi:10.1002/jts.20365

Wang, X. L., Yip, P. S. F., & Chan, C. L. W. (2016). Suicide Prevention for Local Public and Volunteer Relief Workers in Disaster-Affected Areas. *Journal of Public Health Management and Practice, 22,* E39–E46. doi:10.1097/PHH.0b013e31829a303c

Welton-Mitchell, C. E. (2023). *UNHCR's Mental Health and Psychosocial Support.* Geneva: UNHCR. https://www.unhcr.org/africa/media/unhcrs-mental-health-and-psychosocial-support-staff

Wen, X., An, Y., Zhou, Y., Du, J., & Xu, W. (2021). Mindfulness, Posttraumatic Stress Symptoms, and Posttraumatic Growth in Aid Workers: The Role of Self-Acceptance and Rumination. *Journal of Nervous & Mental Disease, 209,* 159–165. doi:10.1097/NMD.0000000000001275

World Health Organization (2012). *Psychological debriefing in people exposed to a recent traumatic event.* https://www.who.int/teams/mental-health-and-substance-use/treatment-care/mental-health-gap-action-programme/evidence-centre/other-significant-emotional-and-medical-unexplained-somatic-complaints/psychological-debriefing-in-people-exposed-to-a-recent-traumatic-event

World Health Organization (2022). Mental, behavioral or neurodevelopmental disorders. In *International Classification of Diseases for Mortality and Morbidity Statistics (11th Revision)* [Online]. Retrieved from https://icd.who.int/browse11/l-m/en#/http://id.who.int/icd/entity/1448597234

Williamson, V., Stevelink, S. A. M., & Greenberg, N. (2018). Occupational moral injury and mental health: Systematic review and meta-analysis. *The British Journal of Psychiatry, 212,* 339–346. doi:10.1192/bjp.2018.55

Woo, T., Ho, R., Tang, A., & Tam, W. (2020). Global prevalence of burnout symptoms among nurses: A systematic review and meta-analysis. *Journal of Psychiatric Research, 123,* 9–20. doi:10.1016/j.jpsychires.2019.12.015

Young, T. K. H., Pakenham, K. I., & Norwood, M. F. (2018). Thematic analysis of aid workers' stressors and coping strategies: Work, psychological, lifestyle and social dimensions. *Journal of International Humanitarian Action, 3,* 19. doi:10.1186/s41018-018-0046-3

Young, T., & Pakenham, K. I. (2021). The mental health of aid workers: Risk and protective factors in relation to job context, working conditions, and demographics. *Disasters*, *45*, 501–526. doi:10.1111/disa.12440

Young, T., Pakenham, K. I., Chapman, C. M., & Edwards, M. R. (2022). Predictors of mental health in aid workers: Meaning, resilience, and psychological flexibility as personal resources for increased well-being and reduced distress. *Disasters*, *46*, 974–1006. doi:10.1111/disa.12517

Building Resilience and Posttraumatic Growth in Individuals and Communities

part III

Therapy and Counselling for Frontline Workers

16

Paul J. Scully

> This chapter is dedicated to Professor Gary Embelton, for revealing the soul in trauma to me.

> *My soul struggles with the memory of her...!*
>
> Paramedic after failed CPR on a child

Introduction

Emergency and other frontline work can be both confronting and remarkably rewarding. Frontline workers often hear people ask, "How do you do this work?" or "I could never do what you do." These workers can, however, struggle with the circumstances with which they are confronted frequently and whilst they generally cope well, they can decompensate emotionally. The aim of this chapter is to outline the authors' personal therapeutic experience having previously been a frontline worker. It will focus on the intensity of frontline work and the brief intimate but at times confronting relationship which can be formed between the worker and the people with whom they engage and will utilize the metaphor of the "Soul" to focus on the personal and intense encounter that can occur in responding to and providing direct intervention in the moment of crisis. Beyond detailing the complexity of frontline work, the chapter will emphasize the necessity for a strong therapeutic alliance by utilizing vignettes identifying different frontline work settings. These vignettes will describe the workers' firsthand experience, why they attended therapy, and the need for the therapist to have an understanding of the nature and complexity of the work setting. The chapter will also refer to the impact on the worker's family, loved ones, and life circumstances.

Frontline Work

Focusing on human behavior and compassion for others, Samuel Oliner (cited in Winston, 2002, p. 363) suggests parental role modeling, learning caring norms, social responsibility, selflessness, empathy, and a sense of

DOI: 10.4324/9781003292807-19

justice as key factors behind entering these professions. More recently, Beyond Blue Police & Emergency Services Report (2018) found that most employees and almost all volunteers across all sectors of emergency work considered their work to be both meaningful and important.

A little-known feature of these work settings relates to the connection which can occur with the people for whom they care or for whom they are responsible. Connection understates the depth of emotional investment which frequently takes place, and how this brief but intense relationship can rattle long-held intrinsic beliefs, views of self, and childhood experiences. Consequently, it can at times be difficult and confronting to provide counseling and therapy for individuals employed in these work settings. It is essential that counselors and therapists have an understanding of the complexity of factors that may surround and impact on workers in frontline intervention.

Therapy, The Soul, and Frontline Workers

The word "Soul" is frequently used to identify the intensity or richness of an experience, or to link an experience to the very core of our being. It can give meaning to an experience and in some instances reveal how distressing or hurtful an experience can be. An early reference to the Soul is recorded in ancient Greek culture; Aristotle held that "the soul is the form or essence of any living thing,"describing the Soul as "the distinguishing mark of living things and the subject of emotional states" (Charlton, 1980).

In a radio show called Ockham's Razor (1998), Emeritus Professor Max Charlesworth was discussing contemporary society. He observed that "we continue to struggle with scientifically and appropriately defining the Soul." Yet the Soul is at the core of many social and religious beliefs; almost all religions attribute the Soul to having certain meaning attached to faith and God, and commonly to define or focus the intensity of the core issue in therapy.

The word Soul appears frequently in daily life: "We need to get to the soul of the matter," "this has been soul destroying," "he is my soul mate." It has also been used formally for centuries as a crisis response: "SOS… Save Our Souls."

A meaningful example of the use of the word Soul is that of soul music, which defines the intensity and depth of meaning behind a genre of music from the early 1920s. Soul music, a popular Afro–American genre, has its origins in blues and gospel music as it expresses the dehumanizing pain of so many.

Frontline workers' experience in the field can sometimes be intense and very confronting. These workers are sometimes reluctant to talk with a counselor as they believe that they (counsellors) wouldn't understand. This points beyond a matter of trust to a matter of safety, security, and connection, in particular when avoidance and "parking" of the experience occurs, until the memory of the incident and the connection to core beliefs and previous experiences becomes too difficult to avoid or starts leading to dysfunctional coping strategies including alcohol abuse or other maladaptive behaviors. In his work examining trauma and compulsive behavior, Briere (2019, p. 14) discussing distress reduction behaviors (DRBs) observed that "people almost always turn to some form of avoidance as a coping response." Avoidance is a common form of coping in frontline workers and brings into focus three key overarching therapeutic factors: the necessity for connection with the worker, the need for an informed understanding of the emotional complexity of frontline work, and the intense and intimate connection which often occurs in a brief but challenging moment when a life is lost or saved or is at serious risk.

In his work, Wallin (2007) observes "viewed through the lens of attachment theory and research, the healing power of psychotherapy derives primarily from the therapeutic interaction." This is especially so when connecting with frontline workers whose emotional vulnerability is or has been at risk. Tedeschi et al. (2018) also suggest that the therapeutic relationship is more important than a particular technique.

Safety and connection, then, are essential components of all therapy and especially so for those in our communities who care for those in crisis as the complexity and intensity of their work require a deeper level of connection and understanding from the therapist. The following vignettes typify the unique nature and intensity of frontline work, and the compelling need for therapeutic "safety and connection" with this cohort.

Alex

Alex was 35 years of age, a tall, thinly built young man with a gentle smile and softly spoken. He was extremely compliant, conspicuously gentle and co-operative in almost every aspect of his interaction with me, and I presume, with others; I could readily imagine his caring demeanor with those he cared for. Alex was married and had one daughter and was encouraged by his wife to seek assistance for what Alex recognized as a significant change in his capacity to relax. In the first session Alex described how he was having trouble sleeping and though he had become used to the shift work lifestyle his sleep and relaxation were now more difficult than ever. He had developed the habit of overcoming his poor-quality sleep by running long distances many days each week; this however was not helping.

We discussed this and various aspects of his work and life, his relationship with his wife, and with work colleagues. It seemed that his life was becoming more "problematic" though he was unclear why. He was experiencing social withdrawal and becoming introverted.

I asked Alex what drew him to the role of emergency firefighter. Alex explained that he had always admired these workers and thought that he could do that work; he also said he wanted to look after himself and look after other people.

Alex was struggling now, particularly when he reflected on cases that were distressing for him. He was reluctant to share this information, let alone the details of cases. I was distracted by his increasing physical agitation, the squeezing of his hands, his re-positioning in the chair, and rubbing his hands up and down on his thighs. I recall being distracted by what Alex may want to share.

I invited Alex to share what was most prominent on his mind. "Well," he said, "I'm sorry to do this to you." He proceeded to share details of an accident in which two trucks had collided. One driver had been trapped for a long period of time whilst emergency personnel worked to free him. Alex found it difficult to tell me even the most basic details of this story and frequently apologized for the tears and other physical and emotional responses as he recounted his experience. He would frequently say "my soul is troubled."

At our second session Alex was able to give more detail about the truck accident. As he did previously, he would move forward on his chair and would rub his hands up and down his upper thighs and squeeze his hands as though he was squeezing water from a towel, again saying he was sorry for telling me this.

Alex explained what had occurred in the lead up to and the cause of the accident but more particularly the fact that he had been on the scene for about one hour which he said "felt like five hours," and that he had established a 'good relationship' with the trapped truck driver. He described his dialogue with the truck driver as workers attempted to free him, and how essential it was for him to continue to communicate with the trapped driver. For the entire duration of the rescue, Alex was not able to see the face of the trapped driver and was only able to touch parts of his upper body to make limited observations about his potential injuries. "But we talked…" Alex said.

Alex was deeply impacted by 'the very personal' relationship which he had established with the truck driver and by his 'being dragged into the private space of this man's life.'

During what seemed like an endless experience with the truck driver, Alex learned how much the truck driver deeply cared for his wife and children. "All he wanted to do was see them and hold them." As time moved on the truck driver had asked Alex if he would survive. Alex struggled to find the words that would neither create unnecessary optimism nor a sense of hopelessness. Alex knew, even with limited capacity to properly assess the patient, that the injuries were serious, and he was at serious risk of not surviving.

Knowing this, Alex, in his softly spoken and caring tone, was able to establish a gentle and positive dialogue with the truck driver. "I knew I had to care for him… a bit like a father." The truck driver gave Alex his wife's name; he also said to Alex "If I don't get through this, will you tell my wife and daughters I love them?" Alex struggled to say these words. As tears gently trickled down his face Alex promised that he would tell the truck driver's wife, realizing that it was essential that he provide some optimism for him. The truck driver passed away shortly after he was removed from the wreckage.

Having shared these details Alex slumped back in the chair and said, "I didn't know how to do this – I didn't know how to say this to his family." This became the moment in therapy in which Alex began to struggle even more; his own childhood experience became 'larger than life.'

Fire service personnel are confronted frequently by death and serious injury, and it is often necessary for them to 'put their feelings on hold' so that they can continue the task at hand. But for Alex, this was a moment of searing confrontation. Alex was conflicted; on the one hand his compelling need to care for and bring compassion and sensitivity to this truck driver, whilst on the other hand realizing that the task the driver had asked of him was "almost impossible for me to do… I was the last person ever to speak with him."

It was obvious that Alex was relieved that he had been able to say these words to me, but he was anxious and apologetic that he had imposed such a burden upon me. In a following session, Alex was again apologetic for his story and again was concerned that this was a burden to me. After reassuring him I encouraged him to talk about what it was that he thought prevented him from being able to convey the affectionate message of the truck driver to his wife.

Thus began the second part of a difficult and confronting journey that spanned several sessions. Though not consciously aware of it at the time of his encounter with the truck driver, Alex was confronted by the trauma of his own childhood experiences and the lack of care.

Alex went on to tell me of the dreadful and dehumanzing behavior of his parent towards him; the abuse was systemic, repeated and with severe emotional and physical abuse and neglect. A poignant moment was when Alex was able to say that "I was not loved. I don't understand love… And I don't know how to give it." He did not trust himself to convey, nor did he understand, how he could convey the love and affection of the truck driver to his family.

This moment brought into sharp focus the conflicted emotional extremes of underlying childhood rage and sadness, and the overtly apologetic, self-deprecating persona all as a result of this intense connection with the truck driver. Referring to childhood abuse and neglect, Ford & Courtois (2013) discuss compromised childhood attachment and suggest that it can lead to long-lasting effects and can influence the way in which people engage with others and within intimate relationships.

Alex had structured his life around controlling his experience of abuse and abandonment. This was not easy, and after many years of frontline work it became the basis for his developing extreme behaviors, complicated relationships, and an ever-increasing struggle to 'push down' the emerging emotional pain. Though it may seem contradictory, Alex chose to work in an environment where he provided care in a sometimes extremely confronting context. Many would find this difficult to contemplate, especially given the context of his background. The intensity of this work, however, allowed Alex to immerse himself in 'crisis,' thus helping him avoid the subconscious pain of his own childhood trauma. As Brown (2015, pg. 17) observes in her work, "[those in] helping professions, first responders, law enforcement officers, clergy, teachers, are populated by people who learned to help others because being helpful and highly attuned to the moods of others was what kept them safe and alive."

Two days after the tragic accident which claimed the life of the truck driver, Alex briefly and courageously overcame his anxiety and visited the wife of the deceased driver and conveyed the loving message to her. The intensity of Alex's childhood experience, the encounter with the truck driver, and reaching out to the truck driver's family had haunted Alex for a long period of time. It had intensified his own lack of parental affection and secure attachment and had now ruptured that which he chose to do in life, save lives and be available to people in crisis.

We all journey in the shadow of our parents. For some this is a guide and a stabilizing influence, for others a torment that continues to lacerate the soul. In their work in dealing with incest and child abuse survivors, Chessick (1978), cited in Pearlman and Saakvitne (1995), observes that the victim may carry a 'soul sadness' or feelings of futile rage. Soul sadness clearly encapsulates the experience of Alex.

Alex, as a *rescuing soul*, was able to act in a way that was the complete antithesis of the experience he endured as a child and adolescent, yet he was able to bring humanity and a rich sense of care and compassion to the truck driver and to many others throughout his frontline career. Ultimately, he was able to step out of his father's shadow, knowing the darkness in his soul.

Tedeschi et al. (2018) point out that emotional disclosure seems effective in facilitating posttraumatic growth (PTG) regardless of different methods used. Following several sessions, Alex began to discover his capacity to be different. He said, "I've decided to work in a different role… I think I can change." He wanted to make a new start in his life.

Mollie

Mollie was a 28-year-old paramedic who was recently engaged to be married when she sought counselling. In our first session Mollie shared that she wanted to make sense of the difficulty she was having with memories of a work incident and also 'some things about my family.' Mollie had worked in a number of locations but said that she had requested to work at and was relocated to a remote area workstation. Mollie explained that when she had worked at bigger stations, male work colleagues would protect her and sideline her in dealing with cases; she felt that her male colleagues needed to protect her in the work environment. "I decided to prove that I was a big girl and capable of doing what I had to do." With some difficulty Mollie was able to disclose, "if I could endure working in a small remote station where I would attend incidents on my own, then I could endure anything." She said that she first wanted to tell me of a case she attended and explain how it had been playing on her mind and had become 'almost impossible to avoid.'

Mollie sat quietly in her chair for some time, and then with her arms tightly folded she began to tell me about a serious motor vehicle accident late at night in a remote area. Initially, she was the only paramedic in attendance. She arrived to find that there were five people in a motor vehicle, two of whom were deceased and three with serious injuries and unconscious. Having called for backup, and initially with only bystanders to assist she described how she was 'in charge' with no one qualified to assist.

"It was difficult…" she said. One of the deceased had been thrown forward and was positioned such that it prevented her from accessing other patients in the vehicle: "…I had to move a dismembered body." After a period of time, a rescue helicopter and two ambulances arrived and transported the three patients to hospital.

Mollie was now the only paramedic at the scene again. She described the exposure to the grotesque images of deceased people; she had never before stayed on scene for such a long period of time. It was almost impossible to look anywhere, she said, without seeing human tissue. She also described the 'mocking and sick' behavior of a number of bystanders. Mollie became angry and wished she could tell them to leave. Information provided later by police informed Mollie that the vehicle had gone on the wrong side of the road and they thought the driver had fallen asleep at the wheel.

Mollie became very tearful at this point. There was a long pause. "I don't understand why I am like this," she said. "I didn't really have control at the scene and I keep getting these thoughts." After another long delay she said, "It's not just the accident. It was what my father said to me and what I had to do to prove myself." I asked her what she meant by 'prove herself.' "I wanted to prove to myself that I could cope and that I am a big girl and capable of doing what I needed to do." I asked Mollie what her father had said to her. With tears in her eyes, she described how her stepfather told her as a teenager to leave home and get a job. "Nobody cared about me… even my real father told me I wasn't worth worrying about. They both treated me like I was useless. From a very young age I was always treated as not worth anything and it got worse when my real dad left; I felt like they destroyed my soul."

Whilst the issues of the traumatic nature of the motor accident were continuing to be intrusive, her underlying anger and shame based on the rejection, neglect, and sense of worthlessness from and caused by her parent and step-parent was pivotal and had become more intrusive. She realized that her strategy to relocate to a remote area where she could have control in her work setting had not worked.

"At the accident I didn't have control… and I felt out of control. Now I'm engaged, will I be a good partner and parent or not?" This experience had heightened her sense of nurturing of others, especially her fiancée, questioning if she would always be thought of as worthless. She also yearned to be a part of her family of origin. The care and support showed to her by work colleagues and fiancée, and her capacity to care for patients, replaced her family of origin, but it confused her emotionally. Mollie felt a need to understand the meaning of her behavior and lifestyle to ensure that the nurturing and affection appropriate for her future family would be nothing like what her upbringing had been.

In her paramedic role Mollie saw an opportunity to "take control and be in charge" but she now was confronted by the uncertainty of her future as a partner, parent, and caregiver. Brown (2015, p. 17) observes that 'because experiences of childhood maltreatment are viewed through lenses created by our many and intersecting components of identity, the challenges we face in creating love and connection in adult life are often flavored by those facets of self.'

Following several sessions Mollie chose to include her partner by sharing her story with him and creating a new sense of meaning in her life. It enabled her to replace her need for control and being in charge with self-care and self-worth; she was not brought up with strong human values in an environment of love and attachment, but she was now able to replace them. White (2004) observed that therapeutically there is a necessity for helping a person reconnect with or reconstruct that which they value in life and validating that person's values and goals for the future.

Sharon

Sharon was a 32-year-old social worker who had worked for several years within a large childcare agency and had moved to a private youth/adolescent care agency. She said she liked working with young people even though it could be difficult. Sharon attended counselling because she said that her partner had become angry with her and left her for a short time because of her drinking and lack of intimacy with him. She shared with me that she was drinking to help her cope. She had become very anxious, having difficulty sleeping and having dreams about a teenage client whom she worked with for several months.

Sharon had grown up in a conservative religious family and was the eldest of four children. She explained that she chose to study social work because of the human values and care which she had learned from her upbringing. Her recent behavior was completely inconsistent with her own standards and she was embarrassed. Sharon went on to say that as a result of working with this client she was having unpleasant dreams which were pushing her to a bad place. When I asked her about the dreams she said, "It's so hard, I failed her I should have done better."

I asked her if she would share her experience with me. "It's not what I ever wanted…" She began to cry. "This whole thing has destroyed my soul… I am a failure… I really cared about her." Sharon composed herself and went on to say:

I had been seeing this 14-year-old girl Tanya for several months, mostly on a weekly then fortnightly basis – she had grown up in a domestic violence family and had been seriously abused at a young age, and was removed and placed in a foster family after having been in a child care facility.

I had worked very hard to establish a good relationship with her, but on this particular occasion, she said that she was being bullied at school and wanted to go to a different school; she was very upset and said that she was having trouble with school work. I had done a lot of work to build trust with her; she told me some details about what was happening with friends who were bullying her now and why she thought this was happening. Because of this I decided to meet with her on a weekly basis in order to ensure that she was coping.

I was suspicious in my following meetings with her that she didn't always share all the details with me; and then it happened… I visited her on a Wednesday afternoon after she had come home from school… She was very upset and in tears most of the time. She said to me 'that she would be better off not being here'… This raised my concern and I spent extra time with her making sure that she would not self-harm. After a couple of hours, I felt more comfortable that she would be okay and she promised that she would ring me if she wanted to talk or if she felt like doing anything to harm herself; I also informed the foster parents of my concern and encouraged them to monitor her carefully. I also texted her during the early evening to reassure her that I was here for her. The following morning, I received a call from the foster parents that during the night she had been cutting herself and had taken an overdose of tablets. They called the ambulance and she was taken to hospital; they said that she was in intensive care.

This was all my fault... and I haven't been able to get it out of my mind. I thought I had been good enough at my work to ensure her safety but I failed; I will never be the same. This is the first time this has happened to me... it has challenged all my beliefs.

Sharon had grown up in an environment in which she learned to recognize the importance of caring for others and meeting the needs of others and then chose to work professionally in an environment in which she could also live these values. Her perceived failure in her work with Tanya overwhelmed her deeply entrenched life standards and values and caused her to 'avoid' by engaging in compensatory behaviors. Briere (2019), discussing distress reduction behaviors (DRBs), observed that people almost always turn to some form of avoidance as a coping response.

In a later session, Sharon revealed that Tanya had, late in the evening on which she harmed herself, received an unpleasant text from a student at school who had bullied her; Sharon did not know of this for two weeks after the incident. "But... I should still have done better."

Brown (2015) suggests wounds heal from the inside out and bottom up. They must be kept open, inspected, and known. Sharon was in avoidant mode for several months and engaged in 'compensatory behaviors' to sustain her avoidance. The pain of confronting her 'perceived failure' was too great. Again, I refer to White (2004; cited in Tedeschi et al. 2018, p. 155), and his observation that therapeutically, there is a necessity for, 'Helping a person reconnect with or reconstruct with or reconstruct that which they value in life and validating that person's values and goals for the future.' This speaks to the core of Sharon's predicament. Of particular relevance is that Sharon not only had to face the circumstances of this experience but also the confrontation of her entrenched and long held values and her commitment to her clients, all of which she believed were compromised because of her perceived failure in caring for Tanya. In his work, Wallin (2007) also speaks directly to this point: 'beyond infancy how we feel clearly remains central to our sense of who we are.' Sharon grew up with rigid moral and ethical religious standards which formed the basis of her values and work standards.

Tom

Tom was a 51-year-old police officer who came to counselling following a long period of poor-quality sleep and what he described as 'shock memories' of a case which he had attended several years previously. Tom was a gentle, softly-spoken person but was obviously not comfortable speaking with a counsellor. He frequently said during our sessions that 'he should be able to cope better than this.' Tom was married and had four children.

In our first session he gave me details of his work history and told me that he had been a plumber prior to becoming a police officer. I asked Tom what it was that persuaded him to attend counselling. He said that his wife Kaye had encouraged him to do so because of his trouble sleeping, and some of the dream stories which he had shared with her; he said it took him a long time to agree to come.

He began to share some details of his work experiences, but as he did, he said that he was not convinced that he could tell some of the details. I asked him why. He said, "It hurts… it still hurts… after all these years."

After a long pause, he began to tell me one difficult story. "What makes this story worse," he said, "is that at the time my daughter was just 12 months old."

"I attended an incident on a construction site; I thought it would be a break in. A major shopping centre was being constructed and extensive groundwork was in progress; the work had stopped due to a serious storm during the previous night. Heavy earthmoving machinery on the site had left large deep track wheel holes in the soft red soil, all of which had filled with rainwater overnight.

Upon arrival I saw workers waving at me directing me where to go; I was shocked to find a tiny child placed on an old towel laying on the ground; the child was wearing only a nappy."

At this point there was a long silence as Tom held his face in his hands. He went on to say that it appeared that the child had wandered onto the site and fallen into a deep truck tyre hole which was full of water. He said, "This is the hard bit. The child had obviously been trying to get out of the very muddy, slippery hole. I can still see the tiny child's finger-marks in the mud around the water hole."

In spite of resuscitation efforts by paramedics and a GP from a practice close by the child died.

"This was very upsetting. I saw this death as a parent. I had my own young children and my daughter about the same age. After seeing this tiny child laying on the ground, I questioned my own ability to preserve life. I asked myself, should I stay in this work? I also got angry with the parents, who lets their child go astray like that? It left a dark spot in my soul. I love my children so much. Long-serving colleagues with more experience provided much needed support to enable me to 'move on,' mostly by talking with each other. They were very understanding and shared some of their experiences… this helped me feel ok."

Tom's experiences of collegial support has been found in first responder research. For example, examining post-traumatic responses in professional firefighters Armstrong et al. (2014) found a sense of connection or workplace belongingness was a significant predictor of PTG. Similarly, in a study of paramedics, organizational belongingness was the strongest predictor of professional quality of life and resilience (Shakespeare-Finch et al., 2014).

In our continuing discussion it became evident that at the core of Tom's response was his anger and frustration at the neglect by the parents of the child. He had mentioned that some of his dreams revealed this. In addition, he said, "There is so much of this going on." Tom knew that I had been a paramedic in my earlier career; he said at this point that this enabled him to tell his story to me.

Conclusion

Frontline work is confronting and at times distressing. I and others have learned many things from these and other clients and are captured by Laura Brown (2015) when she says, "[the client] taught me that before we embrace the power to change our lives as adults, it's sometimes necessary to spend time creating the space to grieve the theft of the opportunity to be a cared-for safe child." This can be difficult for clients but is essential to enable them to move forward.

Not all frontline workers select these professions in response to their lived experience, as was the case in the stories of Tom and Sharon. Those who do frequently find that they are confronted by their inner-soul demons; the impact of repeated tragedy and death and in some cases the circumstances around these events undermine their capacity to cope and may confront their values and beliefs.

These vignettes reveal the emotionally distressing nature of the early lives of some frontline workers and the moment in which their chosen work circumstances shattered their capacity to avoid their pain. But it also "created the space to grieve." Alex immersed himself in caring for others until he had to share love. Mollie looked for ways all her life to have control and meaning and to avoid rejection. Sharon was brought up with entrenched religious standards which meant she could never fail. Tom's upbringing and early life had embodied a deep and enduring commitment of care and respect for others, and thus his anger and hurt at the neglectful parents of a young child.

These vignettes and the lived experience behind them go beyond the "data" that so often informs the therapeutic practices for working with frontline workers. Specifically, it informs the demand for safe connection and attachment in therapy. These frontline workers risked their emotional safety and especially their identity by sharing a story so intensely intimate that they – quite literally – had to bear their souls.

References

Armstrong, D., Shakespeare-Finch, J., & Shochet, I. (2014). Predicting post-traumatic growth and post-traumatic stress in firefighters. *Australian Journal of Psychology, 66*(1), 38–46. doi:10.1111/ajpy.12032

Beyond Blue (2018). Answering the call: National survey on police and emergency services – final report. Accessed at https://apo.org.au/node/206886

Briere, J. (2019). *Treating risky and compulsive behavior in trauma survivors.* Guilford Publications

Brown, L.S. (2015). *Not the price of admission: Healthy relationships after childhood trauma.* CreateSpace Independent Publishing Platform

Charlesworth, M. (1998, June 27). *Ockham's Razor: Scientists and the Soul.* [Radio broadcast] ABC Radio National. Accessed at https://www.abc.net.au/radionational/programs/ockhamsrazor/scientists-and-the-soul/3552164

Charlton, W. (1980). Aristotle's definition of soul. *Phronesis, 25,* 170–186 https://www.jstor.org/stable/4182091

Ford, J. D., & Courtois, C. A. (Eds.). (2013). *Treating complex traumatic stress disorders in children and adolescents: Scientific foundations and therapeutic models.* Guilford Press

Pearlman, L. A., & Saakvitne, K. W. (1995). *Trauma and the therapist: Countertransference and vicarious traumatization in psychotherapy with incest survivors.* WW Norton & Co

Shakespeare-Finch, J., Wehr, T., Kaiplinger, I., & Daley, E. (2014). Caring for emergency service personnel: Does what we do work? Proceedings of the Australia & New Zealand Disaster & Emergency Conference, Gold Coast (QLD), 5th–7th May 2014

Tedeschi, R. G., Shakespeare-Finch, J., Taku, K., & Calhoun, L. G., (2018). *Posttraumatic Growth: Theory, research, and applications.* Routledge

Wallin, D.J. (2007). *Attachment in Psychotherapy.* Guilford Press

Winston, R. (2002). *Human Instinct.* Bantam Press

Community Growth and Resilience in the Face of Disasters

17

Vivienne Tippett and Ben Ryan

Vignette

A small regional newspaper and volunteer radio station has its offices completely inundated by flood waters, losing expensive equipment. The four staff of the business also experience inundation in their personal properties. The valued community information services offered by the business are severely restricted due to telecommunication and electricity interruption. Immediately after the flood waters had receded sufficiently, staff of the business gathered onsite and quickly established the location as a community connection point. Their connectivity in the town allowed them to source available supplies for day-to-day living such as bottled water. In addition, they set up a hot food hub with the support of the local butcher to feed people who were able to return to their homes for the clean-up effort. Over a couple of days, other emergency support agencies such as the Red Cross and Country Women's Association co-located as the area became recognized locally as an informal "hub" – an important focal point for information, social and emotional support and engagement. Locals and regional visitors trapped by the flood spoke frequently about the importance of having access to personal emotional support as well as access to trusted information from reliable sources and an opportunity to talk through what advice about conditions meant.

Community and Resilience in Contemporary Society

How might we effectively define what we mean by "community" in contemporary society? Community has been defined variously as "an entity that has geographic boundaries and shared fate" (Norris et al., 2008); a "group of people with diverse characteristics who are linked by social ties, share common perspectives, and engage in joint action in geographical locations or settings" (McQueen et al., 2001). Community may also be defined on a "case by case" basis, ranging from a neighborhood

DOI: 10.4324/9781003292807-20

to a village, county, or local government area (Sherrieb et al., 2010). Identifying boundaries can be challenging – should this encompass an area where services are provided, administrative borders are located, areas recognized by residents, or a school district? Boundaries are frequently blurred by increased population mobility, communications technology, and relationships between communities and smaller communities coming together in larger groups for some reason, such as faith, culture, ethnicity, or a special shared interest (Mulligan et al., 2016; Sharifi, 2016). Communities are in fact rarely static and so multi-layered approaches are often required to tangibly strengthen resilience. In this context, Sharifi (2016) suggests that a location-based entity could be of any size, from a community to a local government area, and regardless of size an appropriate target for strengthening community resilience.

Community resilience studies have become increasingly common over the last decade as the world faces a shifting hazard profile predicated by climate change. Significant natural hazard events are increasing in frequency, complexity, and severity. However, to date, there has been no single widely accepted resilience model developed which provides direction and support to community leaders and decision-makers seeking to bolster the resilience and sustainability of their communities. In definitional terms, most descriptions of community resilience are based on the seminal work on ecological resilience by Holling (1973). Community resilience is usually defined by the capacity of an individual or group to respond positively to a crisis, the ability to utilize available resources to adapt, survive, "bounce back," and rebuild with or without the assistance of external aid agencies. Resilience is complex and:

> ... the result of a ... set of feedback loops or behaviors that can
> 'balance' the changes created by exposure to an event. The length
> of delay to recovery may be the result of the interactions of these
> feedback loops representing environmental, economic, societal, and
> governance elements.
>
> (Summers et al., 2017)

Consensus on what actually constitutes community resilience is difficult to establish but usually includes concepts such as community leadership, collective efficacy and shared purpose, place attachment, preparedness, and social trust (Cohen et al., 2013; Patel et al., 2017). However, as Koliou et al. (2020) attest, resilience "is not simply the ability to resist or absorb systemic shocks and to rapidly recover from impacts, but also to learn to adapt to future shocks and vulnerabilities." Obrist et al. (2010) drew attention to the fact that resilience should be considered a process rather than a state and proposed a social resilience framework that scaffolded the interactive nature of enabling factors and capacities. Berkes and Ross (2013) integrated principles of socio-ecological theory and developmental psychology in an attempt to further explore the characteristics of community resilience.

Social capital is recognized as a critical factor in understanding community vulnerability and resilience (Straub et al., 2020) across all phases of the disaster spectrum – prevention, preparedness, response, and recovery. Communities are understood to be less resilient and more vulnerable when they are characterized by low socio-economic status; high unemployment or employment in vulnerable industries; high levels of racial, religious, or ethnic division; and a high proportion of older and vulnerable residents (Fraser, 2021). Despite this, where communities have the opportunity to bridge these divides and bond through recognition of shared vulnerability and previously unrecognized shared values, resilience can be fostered in apparently unlikely places (Roque et al., 2020).

Regardless of the theoretical lens applied to defining community resilience, all authors recognize that the contemporary challenges presented by the increasing frequency of major natural hazard events obviously result in significant disruption and failure in key physical and social infrastructure systems. While physical infrastructure and utilities can be repaired, repairing social cohesiveness can be more challenging. This is particularly so in communities where diversity has not been embraced and/or where socio-economic states render some proportion of the community "invisible" during natural hazard events, for example, the homeless or otherwise socially isolated. Where individuals in a community are unable to activate their social networks because they have not existed prior to a major event, how do these communities go about developing a collective reframing of a shared experience and becoming more resilient?

Facing a disaster or natural hazard emergency as a community can result in the creation of new social support structures and opportunities for community connection that may not previously have been known or accessed. There are many examples of situations in which communities have joined together to facilitate immediate support for families and individuals affected by these events. In some instances, these groups have pre-existed the emergency event and have self-activated to support their community. In other instances, new philanthropic groups emerge and self-organize to facilitate access to resources that are perceived to be missing. This phenomenon was well exemplified in the vignette above, in which new awareness of shared vulnerabilities and shared values brought sections of the community into a common space not previously shared. Fostering social, emotional, and physical health in communities by reducing the unnecessary stresses of disengagement and isolation can greatly assist with event recovery.

Social Connection in the Face of Disaster

The increasing challenge presented by social dis-engagement and the degradation of traditional notions of community and connectedness, particularly noticeable in some urban communities, presents impediments to the notion of "community" resilience. Summers et al. (2017) describe resilience as being necessarily underpinned by society and its natural and built environments and risk. Social cohesion is well described in the literature as a protective characteristic of communities that experience growth following significant events and is often defined by communities that have family-centric networks and value structures which include a strong sense of place and social connectedness (Baussan, 2015; Summers et al., 2017).

While metrics exist for the measurement of physical, infrastructure, and utilities risk and resilience as well as socio-economic disruption and economic support post-event, such measures are harder to identify in the context of social cohesiveness, sense of place, and collective growth post-hazard. Work conducted by Boon and colleagues (2012) identified that "the strongest direct predictor of resilience was adaptability and a sense of place." Successful recovery was found to be influenced by financial capacity, family, and neighbor support, and how well they trusted public communication services. The interdependence of social and emotional health and wellbeing with infrastructure and support systems is well understood.

During the COVID-19 global pandemic, social connections influenced approaches at community and national levels. Economically vulnerable populations struggled to endure long-term lockdowns and most countries lacked the ability to maintain a full nationwide relief operation (Ryan et al., 2020). This in turn resulted in different approaches based on community needs and values. For example, in Waco (Texas, United States) the community galvanized together to ensure the successful re-opening of Baylor University in August 2020. There was recognition soon after taking teaching online in March 2020 that the university needed to find a way to safely re-open in the fall of 2020 to assist students, staff, and faculty, as well as contractors and the broader Waco community, to navigate the challenges faced by the pandemic (Ryan et al., 2022). Baylor University was one of the very few institutions which opened for face-to-face activity during this period. The success of sustained activity was due to social connection and the desire of community leaders to tailor their response to reflect community values both during and after the pandemic.

What Builds Community Resilience and Social Growth?

Growing community resilience before and after disasters should be understood to be a process rather than an outcome (Norris et al., 2008). This notion possibly accounts for the fact that there is no single, widely accepted resilience model which provides direction and support for community leaders and decision-makers seeking to bolster the sustainable resilience of their communities. To underscore this point, Sharifi (2016) identified over 30 community resilience assessment tools, all of which have diverse approaches to the challenge. There is however, one resilience tool drawing increased attention and use across the world – the United Nations Resilience Scorecard for Cities. This tool was developed by the United Nations Office for Disaster Risk Reduction with support from the United States Agency for International Development (USAID), the European Commission, IBM, AECOM and other partners participating in the Making Cities Resilient Campaign (United Nations Office for Disaster Risk Reduction [UNDRR], 2022). The Scorecard was first published in 2017 at the Global Platform for Disaster Risk Reduction in Cancun, Mexico and its application has helped to monitor progress on implementation of the Sendai Framework for Disaster Risk Reduction: 2015–2030 by providing a set of assessments that allow local governments to assess their resilience around the Ten Essentials for Making Cities Resilient (UNDRR, 2022). The Scorecard is available in multiple languages and has been applied across the world. New addendums have since been developed which relate to specific sub-categories of resilience, including public health, food security, cultural heritage, persons with disabilities, and industrial and commercial buildings. Clearly, however, a key consideration for the successful application of tools such as this is stakeholder engagement. Identifying comprehensive lists of stakeholders can be a challenging task but will necessarily include representatives of public and private sector agencies, government and elected officials, emergency management agencies, education and public health providers, faith-based organizations, sporting clubs, theatre/art groups, and philanthropic/charity groups. All these agents are vital to support resilience in both individual and community life.

Shared traumatic events do have the capacity to provide opportunities for growth and the establishment of new social connections and shared commitments. Patel et al. (2017) conclude their systematic review by identifying nine consistent elements which characterize those communities which have demonstrated recovery:

- local knowledge
- community networks and relationships
- communication
- health
- governance and leadership that is trusted
- economic investment
- preparedness
- mental outlook.

The Royal Commission into Natural Disaster Arrangements conducted by the Australian Government in 2019 (Commonwealth of Australia, 2020) was triggered by catastrophic fires across several eastern States in Australia. The Commission's report further demonstrated the importance of the collective efforts of the community during both the response and recovery phases of events. Spontaneous volunteering in the face of local events, as occurred in the vignette above, has the capacity to provide a sense of community connectedness and shared challenge: "we're all in this together," but can be difficult to coordinate.

A key challenge for bolstering community resilience is deciding how best to move forward after identifying these shared challenges and areas requiring improvement. Identifying what is needed and how best to address challenges requires wide consultation and engagement with the community. Where this consultation fails, governments and local leaders face significant criticism and resistance. Strategies that are known to assist in this process include impact vs difficulty processes with stakeholders involved in post-traumatic care and support and the wider community engaged to visualize and discuss priority actions according to the impact on community resilience and difficulty (Simon & Cancari, 2012). The Social Determinants of Health theory offers an alternative approach that includes a primary focus on living conditions, work and employ-ment opportunities, and the broader forces that influence an individual on a daily basis such as social norms, economic policies, and political structures (WHO, 2022). This approach also incorporates factors such as lifestyle, education, working and living conditions, healthcare, water, and sanitation (Göran & Whitehead, 1991). By aligning decisions to this framework, all segments of society arguably have their needs and values considered before, during, and after an emergency or disaster event.

Historically community resilience strategies have focused on the various levels of government and public providers, however engaging the private sector is becoming increasingly important as the frequency and complexity of these events outstrip the public purse. In the United States, 85% of the workforce is made up of private company employees. This sector contributes 87% of the country's Gross Domestic Product (U.S. Bureau of Labour Statistics, 2020). In recent years, businesses are examined through the lens of social responsibility (Ketter, 2014) as well as the more traditional commercial success measures. This has led to the establishment of environmental, social, and government (ESG) frame-work which focuses on preserving and conserving natural resources, addressing environmental issues such as pollution, water accessibility, deforestation, human rights, diversity, social justice, laws, and rules and norms for good governance (Ketter et al., 2020). Over 120 companies are currently signed up to the ESG-metrics (World Economic Forum, 2022). In addition to this initiative, the Task Force on Climate-Related Financial Disclosures (TCFD), launched in 2015, provides a process for assessing and addressing climate-related risks for businesses, suppliers, and competitors (Financial Stability Board [FSB], 2017). The TCFD is now also a requirement in the United Kingdom and has been adopted by 2,600 countries across the world (FSB, 2021). Both the ESG and the TCFD provide important avenues for engaging the private sector in addressing community well-being in the face of disaster-related risks and, by association, growing societal and individual resilience.

Summary

Community-led recovery is widely acknowledged in both literature and practice as a powerful strategy for post-event response. Once traditional response agencies have left the area, the engagement of local people in formal recovery roles who are able to activate community energy for the shared return to "usual business" is a very necessary recovery function. Media coverage of the initiative described in the vignette above demonstrated that community members using this spontaneous, informal community hub referenced the positive impact it had on their sense of wellbeing and support in the face of significant loss. In particular, users referenced the importance of a shared sense of place, their commitment to the region and its re-establishment, and the value of "pulling together" in adversity to achieve this. Social and community resilience is a challenging arena and necessarily engages all levels of government, the private sector, and a range of community stakeholders. Success is achieved when the community voices are engaged in all levels of consultation and decision-making across the full spectrum of the Prevention, Preparedness, Response, and Recovery continuum.

References

Antonovsky, A. (1987). *Unraveling The Mystery of Health - How People Manage Stress and Stay Well.* San Francisco: Jossey-Bass Publishers

Baussan, D. (2015). Social cohesion, the secret weapon in the fight for equitable climate resilience. *American Centre for Progress.* https://cdn.americanprogress.org/wp=comtent/uploads/2015/05/SocialCohesion-report2.pdf

Berkes, F., & Ross, H. (2013). Community resilience: Toward an integrated approach. *Society and Natural Resources, 26*(1): 5–20. doi:10.1080/08941920.2012.736605

Boon, H. J., Millar, J., Lake, D., Cottrell, A., & King, D. (2012). *Recovery from disaster: Resilience, adaptability and perceptions of climate change.* Published by National Climate Change adaptation. doi:978-1-921609-63-3

Cohen, O., Leykin, D., Lahad, M., Goldberg, A., & Aharonson-Daniel, L. (2013). The conjoint community resiliency assessment measure as a baseline for profiling and predicting community resilience for emergencies. *Technological Forecasting and Social Change, 80*(9), 1732–1741. doi:10.1016/j.techfore.2012.12.009

Commonwealth of Australia (2020). Royal Commission into National Natural Disaster Arrangements Report. Canberra

Financial Stability Board (2017). Task force on climate-related financial disclosures. *Final Report: Recommendations of the Task Force on Climate-Related Financial Disclosures.* Available at https://assets.bbhub.io/comp any/sites/60/2020/09/2020-TCFD_Status-Report.pdf

Financial Stability Board (2021) *Status report: Task force on climate-related financial disclosures.* Available at https://www.fsb.org/2021/10/2021-status-report-task-force-on-climate-related-financial-disclosures/

Fraser, T. (2021). Japanese social capital and social vulnerability indices: Measuring drivers of community resilience 2000–2017. *International Journal of Disaster Risk Reduction, 52,* 101965. doi:10.1016/j.ijdrr.2020.101965

Göran, D., & Whitehead, M. (1991). Policies and strategies to promote social equity in health. Institute for Future Studies. https://rep ositori.uji.es/xmlui/bitstream/handle/10234/187797/GoeranD_ Policies_and_strategies_to_promote_social_equity_in_health. pdf?sequence=1

Holling, C. S. (1973). Resilience and stability of ecological systems. *Annual Review of Ecology and Systematics, 4*(1), 1–23. doi:10.1146/annurev. es.04.110173.00245

Ketter, W. (2014, June 20). Envisioning and Enabling Sustainable Smart Markets. *ERIM Inaugural Address Series Research in Management.* Erasmus Research Institute of Management. Retrieved from http://hdl.handle. net/1765/51584

Ketter, W., Padmanabhan, B., Pant, G., & Raghu, T. S. (2020). Special Issue Editorial: Addressing Societal Challenges through Analytics: An ESG ICE Framework and Research Agenda. *Journal of the Association for Information Systems, 21*(5), 9. doi: 10.17705/1jais.00631

Koliou, M., van de Lindt, J. W., McAllister, T. P., Ellingwood, B. R., Dillard, M., & Cutler, H. (2020). State of the research in community resilience: Progress and challenges. *Sustainable and Resilient Infrastructure, 5*(3), 131–151. doi:10.1080/23789689.2017.1418547

McQueen, K. M., McLellan, E., & Trotter, R. T. (2001). What is community? An evidence-based definition for participatory public health. *American Journal of Public Health, 91*(12), 1929–1938. doi:10.2105/ AJPH.91.12.1929

Mulligan, M., Steele, W., Rickards, L., & Fünfgeld, H. (2016). Keywords in planning: what do we mean by 'community resilience'? *International Planning Studies, 21*(4), 348–361. doi:10.1080/13563475.2016.1155974

Norris, F. H., Stevens, S. P., Pfefferbaum, B., Wyche, K. F., & Pfefferbaum, R. L. (2008). Community resilience as a metaphor, theory, set of capacities, and strategy for disaster readiness. *American Journal of Community Psychology, 41,* 127–150. doi: 10.1007/s10464-007-9156-6

Obrist, B., Pfeiffer, C., & Henley, R. (2010). Multi-layered social resilience: A new approach in mitigation research. *Progress in Development Studies, 10*(4), 283–293. doi: 10.1177/146499340901000402

Patel, S. S., Rogers, M. B., Amlôt, R., & Rubin, G. J. (2017). What do we mean by 'community resilience'? A systematic literature review of how it is defined in the literature. *PLoS currents, 9.* doi:10.1371%2Fcurrents. dis.db775aff25efc5ac4f0660ad9c9f7db2

Roque, A. D., Pijawka, D., & Wutich, A. (2020). The role of social capital in resiliency: Disaster recovery in Puerto Rico. *Risk, Hazards & Crisis in Public Policy, 11,* 204–235. doi:10.1002/rhc3.12187

Ryan, B. J., Coppola, D., Canyon, D. V., Brickhouse, M., & Swienton, R. (2020). COVID-19 community stabilization and sustainability framework: an integration of the Maslow hierarchy of needs and social determinants of health. *Disaster Medicine and Public Health Preparedness, 14*(5), 623–629. doi:10.1017/dmp.2020.109

Ryan, B. J., Muehlenbein, M. P., Allen, J., Been, J., Boyd, K., Brickhouse, M., Brooks, B. W., Burchett, M., Chambliss, K., Cook, J. D., Ecklund, A., Fogleman, L., Granick, P., Hynes, S., Hudson, T., Huse, M., Lamb, M., Lowe, T., Marsh, J., Nixon, N., Nolan, D., Nunez, G., Matthews, W., Stern, S., Wheelis, M., & Brickhouse, N. (2022). Sustaining university operations during the COVID-19 pandemic. *Disaster Medicine and Public Health Preparedness, 16*(5), 1901–1909. doi:10.1017/dmp.2021.69

Sharifi, A. (2016). A critical review of selected tools for assessing community resilience. *Ecological Indicators, 69,* 629–647. doi:10.1016/ j.ecolind.2016.05.023

Sherrieb, K., Norris, F. H., & Galea, S. (2010). Measuring capacities for community resilience. *Social Indicators Research, 99,* 227–247. doi:10.1007/s11205-010-9576-9

Simon, R. W., & Canacari, E. G. (2012). A practical guide to applying lean tools and management principles to health care improvement projects. *AORN Journal, 95,* 85–103. doi:10.1016/j.aorn.2011.05.021

Straub, A. M., Gray, B. J., Ritchie, L. A., & Gill, D. A. (2020). Cultivating disaster resilience in rural Oklahoma: Community disenfranchisement and relational aspects of social capital. *Journal of Rural Studies, 73,* 105–113. doi:10.1016/j.jrurstud.2019.12.010

Summers, J. K., Smith, L. M., Harwell, L. C., & Buck, K. D. (2017). Conceptualizing holistic community resilience to climate events: Foundation for a climate resilience screening index. *GeoHealth, 1,* 151–164. doi:10.1002/2016GH000047

United Nations Office for Disaster Risk Reduction (2022) *Disaster Resilience Scorecard for Cities.* Accessed at https://www.undrr.org/publ ication/disaster-resilience-scorecard-cities

US Bureau of Labor Statistics (2020). *Spotlight on Statistics.* Accessed at https://www.bls.gov/cps/lfcharacteristics.htm

World Economic Forum (2022). *Stakeholder Capitalism Metrics Initiative: over 120 companies implement the ESG reporting metrics.* Accessed at https:// www.weforum.org/stakeholdercapitalism

World Health Organization (2022). *Social determinants of health.* Accessed at https://www.who.int/health-topics/social-determinants-of-hea lth#tab=tab_1

Summary and Reflections   18

Dagmar Bruenig and Jane Shakespeare-Finch

This book has given the first comprehensive account of trauma, resilience, and posttraumatic growth across a wide range of frontline professional and volunteer occupations and frontline and high-risk work contexts. The individual chapters covering the different occupations and contexts have outlined the core elements of these important work roles as well as challenges and opportunities in providing frontline staff with adequate support mechanisms to achieve high levels of mental health and enhance their capacity for professional and personal growth. A number of things have become obvious across the various chapters, such as how uneven research has been within these occupations. For example, there is considerably more research that has been conducted about the mental health of law enforcement officers and nurses compared to emergency dispatchers and child protection workers. This has effectively silenced the voices of those in the latter occupations. Many of the occupations and contexts covered in this text have not traditionally been included in frontline or high-risk occupations, yet the chapters are very clear that all belong in that category. However, the text is not exhaustive in that regard and it could be argued, especially following the height of the COVID-19 pandemic, that other professions should join this rank, including teachers and pharmacists.

A high level of research with a pathogenic focus has also made it difficult in some areas to identify clearly how growth can be accomplished, particularly in those occupations that have not traditionally been considered frontline workers, such as child protection workers and correctional officers (Chapters 10 and 12). However, the research that exists for all frontline occupations and volunteer groups clearly shows that the picture of posttrauma adjustment is complex and provides opportunities for resilience and PTG as well as negative posttrauma trajectories such as PTSD. This is consistent with research from other populations (e. g., Bonanno et al., 2012; Norris et al., 2009). As has been indicated in the relevant chapters, there is a need to address mental health in proactive (e. g., psychoeducation) and reactive ways from a salutogenic perspective in order to maximize the buffering of negative long-term mental health impacts and maximize the chance for adaptation, resilience, and PTG.

DOI: 10.4324/9781003292807-21

Organizational Responsibilities and Workplace Cultures

Despite varying degrees of research available to explore resilience and posttraumatic growth in frontline occupations, there has been a consistent story around the fact that frontline workers can experience high levels of satisfaction and well-being from their occupations. This is not to minimize the negative fallout from their day-to-day work but rather shine a spotlight on the possibilities to help those that may be struggling more than others.

Workplace culture is one of the central themes coming through in all the chapters as an integral part in a journey to wellbeing, resilience, and PTG. This is also true for those that are volunteering within organizations but are often not really considered as part of an organization (Chapter 7; Chapter 16). In some industries the workplace culture has been described as oppressive (e.g., Chapter 3), or red-taped (Chapter 4; Chapter 10) where a sense of trust is difficult to establish. Nursing research, for example, has shown that a focus away from the overall organizational responsibility towards an individual approach to improving coping strategies is not sufficient to counteract problems of burnout and mental ill-health (Chapter 8). These problems are lessened in frontline occupations where higher levels of trust exist between the workers and management (Chapter 5). Hence, the problem of workplace culture often comes down to leadership as the central issue (Chapter 2).

As Chapter 2 outlined in detail, beyond the organizational culture there is a responsibility to provide early access to programs that support positive mental health in frontline workers. These programs, when tailored to the context and implemented well, also help to foster a feeling of belongingness, supporting attempts to create a better workplace culture.

Motivations for Becoming a Frontline Worker

Motivations for picking up the job of a frontline worker appear to have potentially protective properties in some cultures and contexts. For example, in law enforcement in the USA it was reported that a family tradition of working in law enforcement is a source of pride and practiced resilience as the upbringing around the lived experiences and stories of the elder generation may have provided a buffering mechanism for the younger generation (Chapter 4). This ties in with an understanding of how trust and a feeling of the frontline community being that of family is understood in other frontline occupations as well and does, indeed, attract people to joining as either volunteers (Chapter 7), in professional capacities, or both. In other occupations, however, the motivations might be different. For example, in Australian paramedics, the motivation reported to be behind joining the service was based on a wish to help others, save lives, and have an exciting career. While it is not implied that these motivations are not present in American law enforcement personnel, it needs to be considered how the different impetus for joining a frontline service might hold problems or opportunities for protective mechanisms in these workers. While the chapters on nursing and emergency physicians (Chapter 8; Chapter 9) do not make explicit the motivation behind joining the professions, it becomes clear that the definitions of what it means to be in these professions from the outside, but also from inside, hold difficulties for those workers. It is also clear that providing excellence in clinical care, minimizing physical difficulties, and saving lives is of paramount importance in these professions. The extreme pressures of being there for others that dictate the nursing and emergency physician professions, combined with an expectation to be self-sufficient, provide a fertile ground for mental ill-health that will need to be counteracted by providing prevention and intervention approaches that go beyond self-care.

It may be difficult for a lay person to understand what draws people to professions that require them to be in contexts of constant peril, for example in war zones, camps of displaced persons, or following mass fatalities. In Chapters 11, 14, and 15, we have learned about the motivations for people to put themselves in these positions. They are selfless. In the military (Chapter 11) there is a strong need for people to serve their country, to put their lives at risk for what is perceived to be matters of national security and to serve the greater good. Military personnel are also called upon to assist in times of domestic crises such as following natural disasters, thereby serving their communities. Humanitarian Aid Workers (Chapter 15) seek to assist people in extreme difficulty, displaced from their homes through war or other reasons they flee in fear for their lives and those of their families. In this work context we read of an absolute commitment to issues of humanitarianism, to social justice. In Chapter 14 the authors describe the extreme work context of being part of multidisciplinary teams that are responsible for disaster victim identification. They speak of the challenges of the identification role, both physically and psychologically, and also of the satisfaction they have in providing closure for families who have lost loved ones. Chapters 7 and 17 discuss how communities come together in times of crisis and of the shared experiences of trauma. It also speaks to the capacity of people to help heal individuals and communities through working together. The commonality in all the professions and volunteer roles in this text is one of commitment to the promotion of wellbeing in people and communities around the world.

Global perspectives

We also note that despite strong attempts from the respective authors to provide a relevant, global perspective on the wellbeing of frontline workers, research is predominantly situated in Western cultures with less studies showing research in Eastern cultures, specifically with regards to resilience and PTG. For example, there has been some debate as to how exactly PTG might translate across cultures, in particular those cultures that are different from the West (e.g., Kashyap & Hussein, 2018). As Kashyap and Hussein claim, as well as Tedeschi and colleagues (2018), the concept of positive changes resulting from a struggle with highly challenging and traumatic experiences has been written about for millennia in myths and religions, by philosophers and clinicians. This text has also highlighted that trauma, resilience, and PTG are universal concepts. Yet, there is still a question to be further explored as to how people from different cultures express or experience PTG beyond that which standardized measures capture.

Conclusion

Much work still remains to be done to fully support frontline workers around the world to keep them safe and provide them with a framework that enables well-being and growth. System-pressures such as tight resources and shift-models that are impacting many occupations (e.g., Chapter 8; Chapter 9) will always be present. If the workplace can show compassion and understanding and provide workers with a sense of appreciation, care, and belongingness, much can be gained. Prevention and intervention programs then become believable and deeply incorporated into the workplace culture and can thus show impact in reducing mental ill-health and promoting mental health.

References

Bonanno, G. A., Kennedy, P., Galatzer-Levy, I. R., Lude, P., & Elfström, M. L. (2012). Trajectories of resilience, depression, and anxiety following spinal cord injury. *Rehabilitation Psychology, 57,* 236–247. doi:10.1037/a0029256

Kashyap, S., & Hussain, D. (2018). Cross-Cultural Challenges to the Construct "Posttraumatic Growth". *Journal of Loss and Trauma, 23*(1), 51–69 doi:10.1080/15325024.2017.1422234

Norris, F., Tracey, M., & Galea, S. (2009). Looking for resilience: Understanding the longitudinal trajectories of response to stress. Social Science and Medicine, *68,* 2190–2198. doi:10.1016/j.socscimed.2009.03.043

Tedeschi, R. G., Shakespeare-Finch, J., Taku, K., & Calhoun, L. G. (2018). *Posttraumatic Growth: Theory, Research and Applications.* New York, NY: Routledge

Index